I STILL SHINE

WENDY LAUNIUS

ISBN-10:1-946292-01-X
ISBN-13:978-1-946292-01-8

Printed in USA

DEDICATION

I dedicate this book to Alex, my husband. Also to my amazing children, and to my family who encouraged me to keep on and not give up on myself. I've wanted to let myself go and not push myself many times but y'all have always kept me going and I can't thank you enough. The Facebook support groups that have been so amazing, always there to answer my questions and encourage my recovery. My neurologist, my therapists that have helped me through my journey. My life time friends that have always been there for me. I also want to thank myself for having a second chance at life. I thank myself for fighting to live!

ACKNOWLEDGEMENTS

I am so thankful to be a part if a wonderful group named, " I am a BA/AVM awareness trip". This group has been there for me through thick and thin. During times, I needed support and times I provided my support. Not only does this group help others but it spreads awareness! We spread awareness every chance we get in any way possible. We just started having a yearly retreat for the survivors to meet!

My thanks and appreciation to this group cannot be expressed enough. This group is one of the very informative about what the person may experience after having an aneurysm or AVM. The members of this group have donated their support and good heart and I'm so great full. Without this group, no awareness would reach the outside. People would not have the support they would need.

I need to express my gratitude of appreciation to everyone in the group who have shared their stories and experiences. The entertainment the group provides along with keeping up with the insights on aneurysms and AVM's that maybe mentioned in the news! Without this there would be no reasoning behind this group, I'm so blessed to be a part of.

CHAPTER ONE

When we are young, we just assume 'life goes on'. We do not think about our life ending. Life is all about the now. When we are younger, our world is so small. Even the smallest of things seem life changing, even catastrophic, as though our world is over and we cannot go on. Do you remember those days? I remember so many times that one tiny thing would happens and I would run off crying, locking myself in my room. I was absolutely sure that life was over! You know what I am talking about right? We have all been there. Like that time your best friend in the 6th grade had a crush on the same boy you did, and then you caught them kissing behind the bleachers. Those moments, at that time it seemed as though it was the worst thing that could ever happen! Ah, to be young again...

What would we do if we knew our future? If we knew the date that our life would spiral into the hands of fate, or even worse, into the hands of science. I can tell you now, I honestly would live my life just like a country song. You know the one. "I went sky diving, I went rocky mountain climbing, and I loved deeper, and I gave forgiveness I had been denying." That song, yes, I would live like that. Why do I say that and how can I be certain enough to write in a book that is what I would do?

Sit down a bit and let me explain. I know that because my life did spiral out of my control, and I am living that song every day. I did not know though. I had absolutely no idea.

Life. It's a funny thing. If we knew how it was to play out, I am certain this would be a better world. I know I am a better person. I appreciate life so much more, I love openly and I try not to have any words unspoken. Wouldn't that be a great world?

I am not saying that I was an awful or horrible person before that moment. I was wild, I lived life to its fullest. I had big dreams and the normal teenage rebellion. In some ways, I had a fairy tale childhood, I met my husband and 'knew' he was the one in the seventh grade!

In many ways, I have been blessed. There were times I was unable to say that. Looking back now, I can say with certainty that I have been blessed, and I am exactly where I am supposed to be today.

This is the story of my journey. The good. The bad. The challenges I faced, and the challenges that I still face. All of which has molded me, changed me and blessed me.

~Senior Homecoming~
1996

"Who is that guy?"

Wendy watched the new captain of the football team jog by. She looked at Katie, the newest cheerleader on the team and answered. "His name is Alex, he is okay I guess."

"Okay? That boy is MacPerfect!" Katie sang. Wendy laughed, this new girl was pretty cool.

"Hey Katie, would you want to come to my house after practice and hang out?"

"Ya, that would be great!"

That afternoon they laughed and laughed, shared secrets and somewhere between top roman noodles and Days of our Lives, they became best friends.

"Alex is my boyfriend." Wendy confessed. "We have known each other since the fourth grade. We have been secretly dating, you cannot tell anyone."

"Who?" Katie asked confused as she put the last bowl into

the dishwasher.

"You know, MacPerfect." Wendy smiled.

"The boy that was jogging on the track? That MacPerfect? He is your boyfriend?"

Wendy blushed and shook her head yes.

"Un real! You really are a living that all American girl life, Captain of the cheerleading team dating the hot football star, living in Hoe Dunk Cow Poke Town Texas. Why would you not have said sumthin earlier when I asked?"

"That typical stereo type cliché of the 'All American Teen', It's really not like that. I am going to marry him, he could be the biggest geek in school and I would still marry him. We are soul-mates."

"My mom tells me it's called first love. She said soul mates are not real. She says it doesn't last, the first, second, third. She calls those puppy loves. Kinda like fool's gold, only fools love. Someday, we will know who the real one is she says. When we are older of course."

"The real one what?"

"The one you are really going to marry. That one is called the True Love."

"Well then, Alex is my true love." Wendy smiled.

"Who was you fools love?"

"Alex."

"Alex can't be both."

"Yes, he can, he is my all. He is my everything. He is going to be my husband, the father to our children, and we are going to grow old together sipping tea on the front porch."

"You forgot the white picket fence." Katie teased. "Are you going to the dance after the game tonight?" She asked, gathering her things into her backpack and walked to the door.

"Wouldn't miss it!" She answered. She hated dancing, absolutely hated to dance, she had no rhythm what-so-ever. Despite her distaste for dancing, she would not miss an opportunity to be in Alex's arms.

That night was cool, a little bit more breezy than normal.

Alex was out on the field practicing, for some reason, she had an uneasy feeling about tonight. They were playing a team that was 0-7, there was nothing to worry about she told herself. Wendy smiled and laughed it off, what could go wrong, it a football game like all of the games before and the many more to come.

Wendy could just not get over the feeling that something was not right. It was just a feeling. Everything appeared to be normal, everything was just like every....

"WHOA! We need a medic down on the field!" Wendy heard the announcer yell.

She looked around, she couldn't find Alex on the field or on the sidelines. What was wrong? Was it Alex?

"We are just going to put this around your neck." Wendy heard, she opened her eyes slightly, for some reason that was painful. She could see lights, red and blue lights. Why did that hurt so bad?

She woke up in the ambulance, she couldn't move her head, she had wires all over her body.

"They didn't catch me did they?" Wendy asked the ceiling disgusted that this happened and she could not watch the final game, or more accurately, watch Alex. Almost immediately a smiling paramedic poked his head over hers and smiled.

"Nope."

"They have got to work on that!" She joked.

"They will have time. I am sure the Doctor will not let you get tossed into the air for a while after this one." He winked at her as they arrived at the hospital.

They had just finished taking the CT Scan on her head when her Mom rushed into the room.

"The School is on the phone." He mom said as she stretched the cord as much as she could and handed Wendy the phone. On the other end, she could hear the Vice Principal announce. "The Cheerleader that was injured has gained conciseness and is awake and talking at the hospital." Wendy could hear all the cheers and whistles from the crowd. Her eyes widened as she looked at her mom.

"They are all happy I am okay, it was like really loud

happy!"

"Of course they are dear." Her mom replied taking the phone back. She really did not understand how incredible that moment was to her. She saw the look on her mother's face change.

"What?"

"Alex was injured; he is on his way here. Do not freak, it's nothing serious." The Assistant Coach said as he peaked his head into my room.

Wendy had been trying to hold her breath, hoping the quietness of not breathing would let her hear something, anything about Alex. It backfired of course. She couldn't breath and in the time that she was desperately trying to catch her breath she had missed them rolling him in, and had not heard anything.

It would be accurate to say that was not our night. Silly though, as painful as this was for both of us the night turned out magical and it is one of my best memories of us. Despite the injuries, to me, it was a sign. My other half, my soul mate, could not focus. He could not concentrate because he was horribly worried about me. He felt as though part of him was injured, although he will never admit it. He was so out of sorts, that he delayed and was tackled. He had hurt his foot and had to wait for the ambulance that had taken me to the hospital only minutes earlier, he had to be there with me. We are two pees in a pod!

"Where is he?" Wendy asked the moment her mother opened the door.

"It is a toe. He will be fine. His dad said he is even going to the dance tonight. That is wonderful huh?" She smiled happily thinking that Wendy must be relieved. She had no idea the box she just opened.

Unfortunately, it took the hospital nearly two hours to decide that Wendy's brain was well and all she suffered was a concussion from the fall.

"I want to go to the dance. I promised Alex I would dance with him."

"Absolutely not! You have a concussion. Do you not

realize you are in a hospital?"

"Mom. Please. Pretty pretty please."

Wendy's pleading eyes, pouty smile and dimples were no match. "Fine. If the doctor says yes, one dance. ONE!"

Wendy smiled triumphantly.

Senior Homecoming was a night she would never forget. It was perfect, well except for the concussion and broken toe!

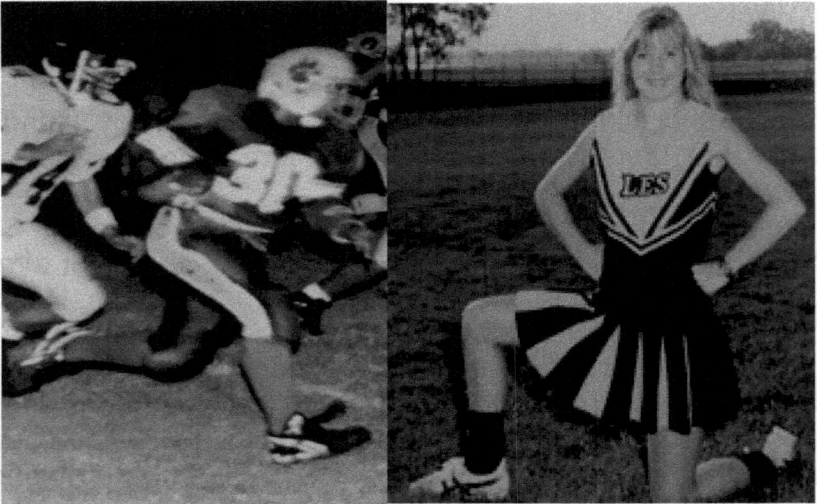

Graduation Day
May 1996

"Stand here."

"Hey you two, let's take a picture!"

Alex and Wendy stopped as they walked out into the grass auditorium and looked at each other, ignoring the commotion going on around them. Alex lovingly smoothed the tassels out on her hat.

"We did it." He smiled

"Today is the first day of the rest of our lives!" Wendy smiled excitedly and pounced a juicy kiss on Alex' lips. She had dreamed of this day so many times. Today was even more perfect than she had ever imagined. Alex standing beside her, holding her hand, made it perfect.

That evening was full of graduation celebrations and food. Lots of food, family and friends.

"Congratulations you two." An unfamiliar lady said to them, interrupting their private moment.

"Thank you, Sue."

"Your Mom tells me that you still plan on playing football?"

"Yeah, we will see. I would love to play for the Cowboys!"

"Wouldn't that be something?" She smiled. "This must be Wendy. I have heard so much about you. I am Sue, I've been a friend of the family before there was a family. That tells you how old I am!" She joked and patted her face as though she was smoothing wrinkles. They all laughed. Wendy liked Sue.

"It so nice to meet you. I am leaving at the end of the month for Galveston. I am going to study Marine Biology."

"Wow, well aren't you the smart one! You got a good girl here Alex."

The night went on with many more conversations. All this talk about their future was leaving Wendy with an unsettling feeling she just could not figure out.

The future, their entire lives before them. A smorgasbord of possibilities. The chance to make your own choices. The chance that she could make the wrong one, was that what was so unsettling?

No, it was leaving Alex. She had not been away from him her entire life. In only a few weeks they would be hundreds of miles apart. That was what was bothering her. Future was here and moving forward, and Wendy was more than aware that there was a part of it she was going to be alone.

Galveston was great. After signing up for her classes, buying books and spending hours in Walmart she flipped on the TV and plopped onto the couch. Tomorrow was her first day of College. She grabbed the new Salt and Pepper shakers she had bought and began to fill them.

Loneliness and quiet surrounded her even though Jim from the evening news was giving a sunny forecast, she felt grey. Wendy reached for the phone to call Alex.

Life Challenges...

"Wendy. Can you please stay and talk with me?" The Professor said as the clock struck three.

She gathered up her papers and stuffed them unceremoniously into her bag.

"Is everything okay Professor Tom?" She asked as she nervously approached his desk.

He handed her the last exam paper. A large red D on the front page.

"Wendy, you are consistently slipping down my grading scale. A couple months ago, you were my star student. Is everything okay? Is there something you want to tell me?"

Wendy was shocked, she did not expect care and concern from college professors. She had always heard from her high school teachers, 'I am not giving you a hard time. I am trying to help you, in college they do not care if you fail.'

"I am pregnant. I am sorry, the morning sickness is not just in the morning. I am getting it under control, I promise I will do better."

"Congratulations on the baby Wendy. I have great hopes for you, you have a passion and I want to see you do well." Professor Tom said as he handed her other assignments he had graded. Wendy did not need to look at the grades. She knew with the D on the exam she was failing the class.

That afternoon she did not go home. Wendy walked around the campus. She watched people, joking and playing tag football in the grass. Everyone seemed as though they had not a care in the world. Why was she struggling? Why was this so hard? She had never struggled before, she was one of those carefree people.

"My hormones need to be committed." She told herself as she finally headed in the direction of home. She needed to talk to Alex.

Wendy waited for Alex to get home. She had been pacing the living room waiting while rehearsing the conversation in her mind. A part of her thought quitting school was the right thing to do, it would relieve the stress. Another part of her thought it was the easy way out, and wrong. She was really torn.

Finally, she heard the front door. Alex had barely shut the door before she blurted out, "I cannot do both."

Alex had no idea what she was talking about.

"Alex, the morning, noon and night vomiting is draining me. I have not slept a good night in months. My grades are falling. I received a D on an exam paper today, a D!"

"That is not the end of the world. There are plenty of preggers in college Wendy, it is not like you're the first one to do it."

"I did not say that I was, however, it is the first time for me, and it is draining me dry."

Alex sighed. He walked over and took her in his arms. "I am sorry. I do not mean to be insensitive. I am sorry this is hard on you. I do not know what it is like to get sick every day."

Wendy smiled, she knew he would understand.

"Can we make a deal?" He asked. Wendy nodded her head yes. "Finish up this semester, I will help out around the house, and help with cooking and laundry, take some of the load off of you."

"Deal." She smiled happily.

April 1998

"*No!*" Wendy screamed at the top of her lungs. "*No!*"

"You have to push! Hold your breath." The nurse was coaching her. "Good. Yes, that's it!" She took her hand. "OK, now squeeze my hand. Push while I count now okay? 10...9...8...7...6...5...4... almost there, keep pushing! 3...2...1... it's a girl!"

Wendy quit pushing and tried to sit up. "Why is she not crying?" She asked as her baby girl let out a whopper of a cry.

"She is a healthy baby girl with great lungs!" The Dr. smiled as he placed this perfect miracle in her arms. Wendy looked over to see Alex take his fingers and gently rub his daughter's cheek.

"I have never seen anything so perfect, except you." He

said as he gave Wendy a kiss. "Thank you."

"Thank you." She smiled. "Sydnee, we waited a long time for you."

When the nurse took the baby to clean her off and weigh her she did not want to let her go. Wendy and Alex could not take their eyes off their daughter.

The nurse placed the identification bands on her ankle, and wrapped her up in a blanket.

"She is a healthy baby girl. She is 19 inches long and weighed in at 8.4 pounds." She said smiling as she finally placed Sydnee back in her mother's waiting arms.

Life was great. She and Alex would both wake up and stare at this perfect little human their love created together every night. Alex held up to his part of the deal. He was working and going to school still.

Final exams were difficult, neither of them had had much sleep and Sydnee was a wonderful distraction. There were many times they would both catch each other just staring at her when studying and they would say out loud, 'back to work', and laugh because they were both guilty.

Summer was coming and Wendy could not wait to go home and show off their little bundle. She had thought life could not possibly get better than it was until now. Being a mother was such a wonderful gift.

It was the best summer of her life. Wendy enrolled in school in September. She was determined to finish.

"I cannot do it. I hate leaving her. I am not doing well in school. I cannot do both. I need to be with Sydnee and give her 100% of me, she deserves that. I cannot be a half time mom and a half time student. I am failing at both of them! I can work part time and we can catch up again."

"I know. Wendy, I will provide for my family, if it is the money..." Alex said. Wendy could tell that his feelings were hurt. "We are just so close, there is only one semester left."

"We will finish, just not now. Let's move to Houston, we can get a small place, they have good hospitals, and we will be closer to home."

Is this not home?" He asked. "Wendy, why are you doing this?"

"I have told you why Alex. Houston is big, I need to be in a city if anyone is ever going to 'discover' me. Look at Anna Nicole. She got out of a small Texas town and now she is famous." Wendy shut the lid on her over stuffed suitcase. Grabbed the handle of the other and flung it onto the bed that she quickly began to fill. "I am going to be famous like her. We are a lot alike, you know that?"

"Alex, Houston is not that far from Dallas, and when you get on the Cowboys team, we will move."

"I do not want you to have to work two or three jobs. I want to see you every once in a while, and after the baby comes you need to have bonding time. You cannot be working all the time just trying to keep us fed. We are partners, we should do this together."

"You win. If it is Houston you want, we will move to Houston."

Wendy kissed him and smiled. "Thank you."

"One condition though," He smiled his wicked grin. "We will finish school."

"Deal." Wendy said as she reached over to give him another big kiss. "Thank You."

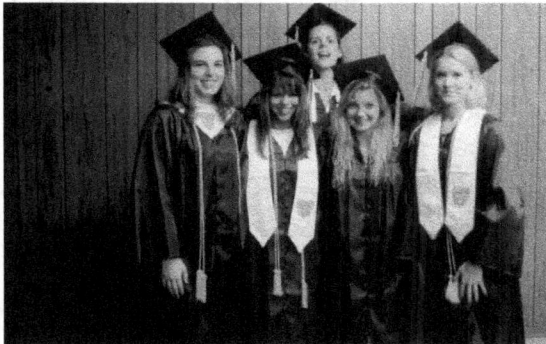

Graduation 1996

CHAPTER TWO

HOUSTON 1998

Houston was everything that Wendy thought it would be and more.

Sydnee was growing so fast, she was the smartest baby ever born Wendy thought. She started eating solid food when she was only ten months. She was crawling at ten and half months and running around the living room not long after.

Like every new parent, Wendy and Alex baby proofed everything. Every door had a plastic 'cannot enter' even though Sydnee was years away from reaching door knobs.

It was not long before life had another surprise in store.

"Alex." Wendy said as she walked into the room. Alex was watching a football game. Normally, Wendy would not interrupt a football game, but this was important.

"What? Can this wait? There is a minute left, they could win it on the field goal." He said not taking his eyes off the television.

Wendy smiled walked over to the remote and pushed the power button.

"What are you doing! Wendy! Turn it on! I am going to miss it!"

As Alex was about ready to have a conniption fit, Wendy handed him the stick she had in her hand.

"Don't touch anything but the handle, I just peed on it." She said as Alex threw the EPT stick down as though it had just burnt him.

Wendy laughed and picked it up. Showing him the positive stick.

His eyes widened. "Is that?"

"Yes." Wendy beamed.

"We are having another baby?"

"Yes, do you remember the fourth of July?"

"We are having a baby!" He screamed as he lifter her in the air and spun her around, completely forgetting about the football game.

April 2000

"I am really worried about your health and the babies." Dr. Jones said. "I think we should induce, your both showing signs of distress."

"No! Doctor please, let me carry her a little longer."

"Do you understand that at any time something could happen, you could lose the baby or even your life."

"They cannot have the same birthday. I do not want that."

"Two weeks, I want to see you next week though."

Wendy looked down at her swollen belly. "Do you hear that baby? You can stay in there until after your big sissy's birthday."

Believe it or not, the baby waited. One week after Sydnee's second birthday they welcomed their new daughter.

Alyssa was a tiny flower that weighed in at 5 pounds. She was small but strong.

October 2000

Wendy through fifteen fashion magazines and two packages of diapers in the shopping cart. And grabbed the Dallas Observer and the Houston Chronicle, she wanted to find a part time job.

When Wendy got the girls down for their nap, she spread the magazines out on the table and started to read the one with the article about Anna Nicole. She was going through a court battle with her late husband's family.

There was a knock on the door.

"It's open." She yelled.

Heidi walked into the kitchen, chewing her gum loudly. She was a firecracker, always energetic and carefree. Wendy was so glad to have met her and that they quickly became friends.

"You need to tell that man of yours that you are going to Dallas this weekend with me."

"That is not going to happen." Wendy laughed. "Did you see this? Can you believe that she has to go through this? I feel so bad for her."

"Why? That girl is a gold digger."

"You do not know that, no one really knows. She was there for him, and she did take care of him. Who knows what kind of arrangement they had." She said defending Anna Nicole.

"Okay, what-ever. You have to go to Dallas with me! Please!"

"What is so important in Dallas?" Wendy asked.

"It's amateur night."

"Amateur night for what?"

"Dancing. The Kitty Kat Klub"

Wendy laughed out loud. "I cannot dance hunny, you are on your own. Wait! The Kitty Kat Klub? Is that a strip club?"

"Yes, your Anna Nicole got her start stripping so do not put it down."

"She was a model. That is what I want to do, I want the world to know my name, just like her. I have even been practicing my walk. Watch!" She said as she got up and did her best catwalk impression in the kitchen. Wendy tripped and burst out laughing.

Heidi laughed. "I can tell you have been practicing. Oh Wendy, please go with me. I cannot do this alone. Who knows maybe there will be someone there that has modeling connections. It's not what you know, it is who you know."

She was right and Wendy knew it. The next few days she begged Alex to watch the girls so she could drive to Dallas. Surprisingly, he agreed. He had told her she deserved some girl time.

She felt bad for not telling him exactly what they had planned in Dallas. She had her yes, and she knew that would change if she told him the complete truth.

~AMATURE NIGHT~
Dallas Texas 2003

Dallas was a fourty-five minute drive from League City. Shelly was high on energy drinks spiked with Vodka.

"I cannot believe we are going to do this."

"Oh Wendy, thank you! I could not have done this without you, even the vodka does not give me the encouragement that you do."

"I may take a swig of that energy drink."

Shelly handed her the Monster can. Wendy pushed it away. "I am driving!"

"Okay, if it makes you feel better, I will go first. You will be a hit after me, your looks are to die for!"

"That is sweet. You're a ten Shelly, do not put yourself down. They are lucky to have us both!"

"That is right. They are going to beg us to dance full time."

"I do not know about that. If Alex found out about this. Oh, my gosh, I do not think it would have a good ending."

"That man loves you so much. There is nothing that you could do that would change that."

"Rob a bank, commit mass murder, or strip. I think that would change things."

They both laughed. "Maybe mass murder. If I robbed a bank, I am pretty sure he would make me return it and beg forgiveness. I doubt he would rush down and file for a divorce. We have girls, he needs me around."

CHAPTER THREE

I believe one of our toughest struggles had to be when I decided I wanted to be an adult entertainer. Yes, a stripper, as many people call them. Having been an entertainer for years, and to toot my own horn, I was pretty good at it. That may not be something some people would think is 'bragable' but I am not ashamed. This profession built my confidence and help me get into the modeling world. I can never judge any woman who works in this world. I know the ups and downs, the stigma that comes along with the job and I am grateful for the experience of being a part of it.

I know all there is to know about this profession, the real life of being an adult entertainer- not the fictional world you see in the movies. I am sure things have changed through the years as everything does. Some may not think this a good thing, but I was able to experience a lot. I have been cursed out by wives and harassed but then I explain to them-this is my job, I am not your husband's keeper. Most of them would understand and go on their way to no doubt put their husband in the dog house.

The best memory of my past profession, I was called into the office and asked if I was interested in doing a photo shoot for a bill board. I couldn't believe what I heard, a billboard? How many people get to be on a billboard! Of course, I did it and that was my first step into modeling! It was such an amazing experience I will never turn my back on this profession or look down on it, even if it is controversial.

I cannot complain about being an adult entertainer. I have met the most wonderful people, and they do not judge others. We became a very close group of girls who I now consider to this day family. Despite what you may believe, a number of us became models. Some of the younger girls would come to me for advice, on how to advance into a modeling career. That was something I felt proud of, to help aspiring models felt great!

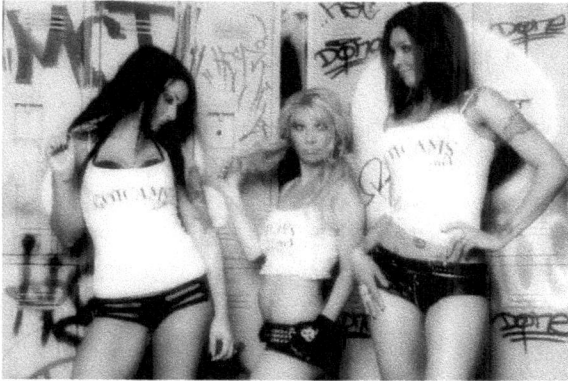

As I followed my career down the road of adult entertainment, and the modeling industry I began to attend casting calls to movies. I was extremely nervous on the day of my first casting call, I was actually shaking! I had no clue what to expect. Come to find out they were like model gigs. They tell you what they are wanting, ask you if you have any experience, why you want that part and then they give you a few lines to say to a table of people who you have no clue who they are.

I had gone to at least seventy casting calls before I got my first callback! Well it happened to be a roll where they wanted me for one part and my friend for another! How lucky is that! I accepted the role without even giving it a thought. Almost immediately we started having group meetings with the cast and crew. I must admit it was so much fun, and an experience I feel grateful to have experienced.

I was told by the writer, who had chosen me for that certain role, that she wanted me to play that Brittney Spears, before the head shaving incident, she was the all American girl whose dreams come true, and in great shape! She had the perfect hair, abs, legs, thighs and of course the butt. Like any woman would do, I told my husband Alex what she had said. I was lucky enough to have a work out guru for a husband, I was married to the best personal trainer I knew. I wanted him to get me into shape, perfect all those areas that the writer had mentioned, form myself into this character. I was already thin, and had abs so that wasn't a concern. No, I needed some help on toning. Alex was not exactly thrilled but he knew I would not take no for an answer.

We started the next day. I did squats, walked, ran along the nature walk and the rolling hills. I gave it my all even when I wanted to give up, I was determined.

To my complete shock, I got another call from another writer. This time they wanted me to play a role for a documentary! I couldn't believe it! Two roles, Two movies! One a horror movie, and the other a documentary.

I now had two reasons to get into perfect shape. Let me make this very clear, I took this very seriously and it was a grueling, never ending challenge.

I received the script for the horror film. Wow what a feeling to have your first movie script. I cannot even explain how surreal just staring at the words on those pages felt. This was really happening for me.

I studied my words hard and continued my training sessions. It wasn't long, I had the documentary script and was studying my line for it as well. My world was looking wonderful. my life time dreams were coming true, finally after all the hard work that I had been put myself through to get here, it felt good. It was an amazing feeling. I wasn't doing all this for just me, I wanted to make my family happy. I did not want to have to keep struggling. I did not want my children to struggle. We all want to provide for our families and give them a better future. I wanted what we all want, a good life for my family. I was doing that, and I was almost within reaching distance of it.......

That all changed in one night. My life was about ready to take on a role of its own, one that could have been written for a lifetime movie. The characters in this script were real though, real doctors, real blood and real pain with a possible real death scene.

CHAPTER FOUR

In the Blink of an Eye
June 23, 2013

Wake up! Wake up! Wake up!" A voice was shouting in my head. It was an urgent voice that startled me. I opened my eyes in a panic. What was happening? I must have been in an accident.

My head feels as though it is in a vice-grip, this pain is something I had never experienced before. Giving birth did not even compare to this pain. I must have been in an accident I told myself again. I tried to ease the pain by crushing my head between my hands, it did nothing.

"Something is wrong with me." I said to myself as I stumbled out of bed. Everything around me is spinning, I cannot seem to get my balance.

As I stumbled down the hallway and out the door all I can focus on is the pain. Where am I. Where am I going?

"Wendy, are you alright?"

My neighbor is looking down at me. I look around, this is not my house. Where am I? What on earth is wrong with my head?

"Go get Alex!" I heard my neighbor Heidi yell to her husband Romeo.

"He is at the door." He replied. In a haze, I looked over towards the door and saw Alex walking towards me.

"Wendy! Look at me! Did you take something? What is

wrong?" I look up at Ann, shaking my head no. Wait. I remember, I took an allergy pill. I try to speak, but the words will not come out. Why can't I speak?

Alex took my hand as he sat down beside me. He is questioning me. I cannot speak! Tears fill my eyes. The pain from thinking is too much. Everything starts to spin, I feel as though I am going to vomit, then everything went black.

I open my eyes to a horrific pain. The gurney is being latched into place inside the ambulance.

"She overdosed." The paramedic was saying. "We are taking her to Clear Lake Regional."

"No, I know my wife! That is not it, there is something wrong!" I hear Alex argue with this strange voice. Desperately I try to open my eyes. I can see flashing lights, hear the panic in the voices around me. The struggle to focus is too much, it is too painful, I once again slip into the darkness. It does not hurt in the darkness I tell myself...

2:30AM- Clear Lake Hospital waiting room

"Launius Family" A doctor called into the waiting room of the hospital.

"Here." Alex said as he rushed over toward the doctor. It had been only an hour since they took Wendy in for imaging, it had seemed like an eternity.

"I am sorry. The tests show that your wife has suffered a brain aneurysm, there is extensive bleeding in her brain. She needs to surgery immediately if she is going to survive." The doctor lowered his head. "We are not equipped for this type of trauma. She is being prepared to be transported via life flight to West Houston Medical as we speak. They are a trauma center, they are equipped for something like this, they have great doctors. I have already contacted a neurosurgeon, he is one of the best. He is waiting."

"What does this mean?" Alex asked confused. "Is she going to be okay?"

"I really cannot answer that; you should talk to the neurologist." The Dr. said sympathetically. From the look on his face, Alex knew the outcome could be grim.

He felt as though the bottom of his world had just given

way. "I need to go pick up my children. I will meet her there." He said as he began dialing Wendy's parents to give them the devastating news. Alex took a deep breath as the phone began to ring, this was not a phone call he ever wanted to make.

As Alex drove home to pick up his daughters, a fear consumed him like never before. Wendy was lying alone in the hospital, her life hanging in the balance. The balance of what he asked himself? Memories began to flash before his eyes. Wendy in the fourth grade, she was the new girl in school. She had taken his breath away at ten years old. She was wearing turquoise boots with tassels and a jean mini skirt. She had the smile of an angel. At that moment, his heart belonged to her, he knew then, she was the one. The birth of Sydnee and Alyssa. The horrible birthday cake she had botched on his 18th birthday, that tasted like flour. Their first kiss, the memories flooded his eyes with tears.

Would they make more memories together? What about the girls, they need their mother! He was numb. What was he supposed to tell the girls? Sydnee was fifteen, Alyssa was only thirteen. They needed her more now than ever.

Alex finally arrived home, the girls were next door at the neighbors. They were great people, they were like parents to them and grandparents to the girls. He was grateful that they were there for the girls right now.

He knocked on the door.

"How is Mom? Where is she?" Alyssa cried.

"Sit down." He answered.

Romeo could tell by the look on his face, he gave Alex a pat on the back in support. Telling the girls was one of the hardest things he had ever had to do. He could not help but ask himself if this was the first of many more to come.

"I have never lied to you girls. I am not going to start now, I wish I could and tell you that Mom is going to be fine, but I honestly don't know if she is going to be."

"What is wrong? She took too many allergy pills right? I saw the pills on the counter." Sydnee cried, desperately hoping this was just a simple mistake and life would go back to normal.

"No Sydnee, the doctor said your Mom has had an aneurysm. It is blood vessel in her head that is bleeding. They are sending her to West Houston. The doctors are going to do everything they can to try to help her."

He had never cried in front of the girls. For the first time, they cried together and they got down on their knees and prayed together.

Alex and the girls arrived at the hospital before the helicopter. They watched the doctors and nurses unload her. There was so many wires, tubes and machines. She looked pale. Alex knew he had to be strong for his children. On the outside, he put on his Dad face. On the inside, he was falling apart. Asking himself over and over, how do I live with half a soul?

That night changed all of our lives forever. Rather than being in the movies, I felt as though I was living in one. It began playing out as a real tear jerker. A woman who is struggling to make it big in Hollywood, finally gets her big break. Suddenly her world comes crashing down when all her struggles are ending, and her dreams turns quickly into nightmares. Yes, I was living the leading role in a Lifetime movie.

I will never be on the same course, my struggles are different, my dreams are not set as high on Sunset Blvd. as they used to be. I am not the same person that I was that day, I am this character I really do not know. I am learning the new me, and I am getting to know who I am now a little bit more every day.

This movie seems to have no ending so far. Like the 'song that never ends'. Of course, this is how it feels to me. It's my life. My dreams are dead, it all ended in the blink of an eye. I am gone, I am in the same body, I am the same, yet I am a complete stranger to myself. I long for the person I was, yet I have happily buried her. I hate the person who now breathes in my body, yet I embrace her with love and pride. She is a survivor.

Survivor, that is a word that has taken on an entire new meaning for me. To me it was twenty contestants fighting, lying and competing to be the last man standing alone on an Island. What a great show! I have watched it from the beginning, even thought to myself I could win that, I could be the survivor....

Um hello? God? Umm I think you misunderstood, I wanted to be the survivor on a tropical Island and win a million bucks.

Even without the million bucks, I am a Survivor. I beat the odds. I have insight! I know what matters, who matters. I know I am strong. I appreciate life, family, friends, moments, but most of all, I appreciate the morning sun. I am grateful for life in ways I never would have been.

Like I said earlier, we do not know what the future holds, if we did, do you think it would change you? You cannot predict the future of your spouse when you both decide to take that vow. No one can see what the other will encounter. Who worries about Arteriovenous malformation, better known as AVM or a brain aneurysm.

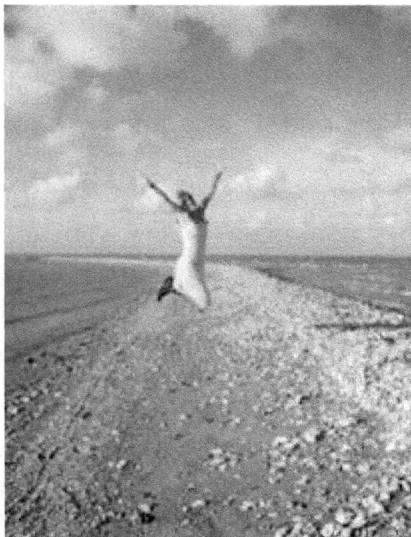

CHAPTER FIVE

Behind the Scenes

The situations a spouse goes through are extremely hard on them. The demands of each family member are crucial to the family's survival. The duties of each member of the family is changed forever. My family has and is going through this.

Our extended family doesn't really see the struggles that my husband and kids are going through, unless they are our parents cause of course, we talk to them about what's going on. Relatives don't realize the hardship. Like two incomes down to one, oldest daughter taking on a job to provide for the family, our youngest struggling through every day teenage life.

This is all hidden from other eyes. It's not their burden to bare.

One night, in 2013, I awoke with a massive headache. When I got out of bed I had no balance, and I kept hearing voices say, "get up, get up!" I kind of snapped awake like somebody had shocked me and I remember that it scared me a little. For a moment, I thought I had been in an accident. All I could say was, "something's wrong with me." I couldn't walk right, I was unstable. For some reason, I went to my neighbor's house, hoping they could help me. I sat on their couch and quickly became extremely sick. I couldn't stop vomiting. I'm so happy my husband, Alex, was there with me. The next thing I recall is that I blacked out.

At the time this happened I had been working on learning

my lines for both movies and working out to get that body every girl wants. My lifetime dream was coming true. I wasn't doing anything hard or stressful at all, although I did have everyday stress like everyone else. Everyone knows those headaches that come with that stress. I also had allergies, and that day I had taken three over the counter allergy pills at 7-8pm so it wasn't the medicine.

The emergency crew that showed up had thought I was overdosing. They took me to the closest emergency room. Not long after I had arrived, the Doctors told Alex, my husband, that they had to care-flight me to another hospital because I was having an AVM, a brain aneurysm. Alex went home, he got our children from our neighbor's house, and told them the news. He was so worried he also beat the care-flight to the hospital.

An AVM is a very rare brain aneurysm. They told Alex to call our family. I was not expected to live. The doctors performed emergency surgery on me, and now I am called a miracle. At that time 4 others came in with aneurysms, but sadly, none had survived. My brain aneurysm was so unique, by all accounts, I was not supposed to live.

They shaved my bangs and the hair above the back of my neck. They placed a tube in the front of my head in my bang area. I was unconscious for a few days. I don't remember any of this. All of this was told to me or I read it in the daily journal my family kept while they kept vigil in the hospital.

I eventually gained consciousness. Giving signs when asked, I would move my toes, small things like that. Eventually, they removed the tube because I kept trying to pull at it. I didn't like it obviously. They even tied my wrists to the sides of the bed, like I was in an asylum. I was excited when they decided to not do that anymore. I suppose I had learned my lesson.

So many people came to visit me while I was still in the hospital: my high school best friend, my sister and my step-sister, my model friends, some Dr.'s, and the care flight crew.

One question I'm asked often is did I see or experience anything while I was unconscious. Well I did! My grandma and uncle who have passed a while ago visited me. They would walk around the corner into the room, and my grandma would hold my hand while my uncle messed with the machine I was hooked up to. My grandma would put her fingers to her lips and tell me, "Shhh." Then my uncle would put his hand on my grandma's shoulder, and as quietly as they came in, they walked out. I'm told the alarms on that machine would go off often and the nurses came in to check on me and that machine. So I'm thinking my grandma and uncle were making that machine go off on purpose.

When my family was gone and no nurses were in my room I was left with nothing but that wall and that ceiling with those ugly dots on it. I think I made a maze out of them a few times. Thoughts ran through my mind like clockwork. Wondering if I was ever going to be a good mom and wife again? Is my modeling career over forever? Will I ever be pretty again? Will my family look at me different now? Will my family love me the same?

My family would stay overnight with me, having to sleep on that cold hard floor. I feel so bad that they had to do that. I also remember the hospital had me on way too much medicine. They were overdosing me so bad I couldn't keep anything down. I expelled everything I ate because of all the medication they had me on. I also became more constipated than I already was. Finally, my family noticed that they had me on way too much medication, so they said something to them. As soon as they took some meds away, I became better. Being constipated was no fun, if you ever had to experience an enema you know what I am talking about.

After a while I'm not sure if they had given me something to help make me go but I couldn't control the urge and as embarrassing as it sounds I messed myself a dozen times. My loving family and a few of the nurses cleaned me up every time this happened and I can't thank them enough. That is so embarrassing still today. But I couldn't help it I understand. I'm just so thankful my family and nurses understood.

Let me tell you, I do not like chocolate pudding or apple

sauce anymore! The pills they gave me were so big, my family had to crush them and put them into the pudding or apple sauce, so now I can't stand those anymore. I spent the 4th of July in the hospital and got to hear the fireworks show that Houston put on. I called them "boom booms"!

They didn't waste any time starting therapy. The physical therapist put a large belt on me that looked like it belonged on a straightjacket, and huge yellow socks that had nonslip grips on the bottom on them (not stylish), and put my hands on a walker. No words can explain how hard it was to just take one step. A voice inside kept saying "you've come this far don't give up now." I wobbled like a penguin, not far but as far as I could, then I headed back to my bed. That would wear me out. The endurance I once had was no longer with me. I was given a wheel chair that I could not wheel around because I just wasn't strong enough.

The first thing my therapist had me remember and do every day until I got back into a routine was brush my teeth! I remember crying over the sink in the hospital room and she comforted me by telling me a poem I'll never forget, the famous poem, "Footsteps". The famous poem about Jesus walking on the beach. I don't know why she chose that poem but it comforted me.

Next, she taught me to put on my shoes. She gave me special laces that were curly and I didn't have to tie them like normal laces. My speech therapist had me repeating words and finishing sentences, singing little rhymes. Sounds weird but singing is the best therapy. Till this day I now sing in the shower. A song my grandma would sing to me. All of that is what my day, each day, at the hospital consisted of.

I was in the hospital for 3 months. My recovery was long, and still my journey continues while I'm home. I got to go home with the wheel chair and walker. I also had a catheter, no fun what so ever! My mom bought me a cute stylish bag that the catheter could go in and we could tie the bag to the walker so it wouldn't be such an eye sore.

Being so young, having a walker and a catheter is overwhelming and embarrassing. People look at you with judging glances, young people asking their parents what happened to get that, then more stares from the parents, the whispers. They think I can't hear them. I can and I might not show it but it hurts. I just kept my smile on and kept moving on. Cry on the inside, smile on the outside.

When I was discharged, my parents suggested that I stay there until we get stable again and are able to find a home/apartment down here in south Texas again. This effected our living situation enormously.

We went from a double income family to one. I had our two girls with me at my parent's house, my husband had to sell all our belongings so we had money. A whole house full of furniture and memories. He packed what he believed were most memorable to us and the girls. After that, he sold everything including washer, dryer, bedroom furniture all for $500, not much. Dogs went to my neighbors and he brought the cat since she is very old. $500 couldn't even buy a couch these days. He didn't have a choice, he was determined to be with us at my parents and it was driving us both crazy being apart.

Finally, we were once again all together. We lived on my Parents farm in a small cabin. When I say small, I am not exaggerating, there was barely enough room for everybody. I continued therapy while I was there, determined to get better. It paid off. I did have to go to the ER often for the UTI's due of the catheter. I finally found a urologist and he got me off the catheter! Eventually, Alex had to leave to back down south to get his job back and find us an apartment. This was hard, he was, and still is my shoulder and my strength.

While he was gone, my mom cooked everything she could to put weight back on me. I was down into the 80's, not good. I slowly gained and I was urinating on my own! I liked to go outside and watch the horses, cows, and donkey. They were like therapy. I just enjoyed watching them while they were in the field. It is a proven fact, there is something about healing and animals. It saddens me that this is not a common practice in rehabilitation.

I would take my walker outside and practice walking with it. I would walk tree to tree, dodging cow patties, and that was a huge therapy. I got good at moving the walker around. Sometimes, I got brave and put my walker to the side and try to walk without it, finding the closest tree possible. Not realizing how far I would get going tree to tree, I would look back and say, "Oh crap" I would turn around and head back to my safety net, the walker. I got good enough to where my grandpa noticed, and he made me a cane.

He got one of his old golf putters and put a rubber bottom on it, and I used that as a cane. It meant so much to me, his care and dedication while he was thinking of me and making me that. I had to get used to it. It was hard, but it was therapy!

Eventually, Alex got his job back and got us a 2-bedroom apartment in League City, TX! We moved into it having to start all over without having a couch, or even beds. My parents had bought us beds while we lived with them, and we had a recliner that my sister had given us. Christmas was easy for me to tell everyone what I wanted. I wanted everything for our apartment, of course!

Under one income, my oldest daughter had to work to help out. This was not an easy decision. She got a job working at Little Caesars Pizza. With her working while in school, responsibility took away her fun times: no hanging out with friends, no movies, no activities, not anything teenagers enjoy. This tore us up as parents.

My youngest was not doing well in school, her grades fell and soon she was failing classes. Soon after that, our oldest daughter's grades followed. Her dyslexia was getting better, but her grades were not. She worked more hours pushing herself to the point where she couldn't make up her grades. My youngest went to the dark side, I guess you can say, her clothes were black all the time and long sleeves no matter if it was hot or cold. As the year ended we found out my youngest was harming herself.

My oldest was being harassed by her boss in inappropriate ways. Not what any parent wants for their children, horrible first year back on our own. I think the only good thing is being back in League City, close to Galveston, which I love dearly. We made our oldest quit her first job, and my youngest decided to stay with my parents and be with her horses. We are hoping they will cure whatever she maybe going through. I blame my AVM for all this. I blame myself.

So now it's two years since my AVM. I'm doing as well as can be expected. Alex is now supervisor! He takes me where I want to go, if we can afford to spend a few dollars, I go to Galveston to walk on the beach often, and I love this feeling. I like to visit the hospital and walk down the hall that we call "sky bridge" because I used to not be able to walk it all. Now I can!

Loud noises bother me, like motorcycles and sirens. I experience flash backs of my recovery and I ask Alex if they happened or not. He's my "go to" guy for answers. Since my AVM, we've had deaths in the family. Alex's uncle and cousin have passed away, and that is hard for me to handle. I cry a lot now, I can't help it. Also, my grandpa has passed away. He was my favorite cowboy, my side kick, the one that *silently watched me.* His death still gets to me. I know, more than most that death is a part of life, I understand that more now. I understand death so much more than what I did before. I was blessed to get many possessions that were my grandpa's, so our house is now a home. We no longer live in a 2-bedroom apartment. We are now living in a 3-bedroom home, looking to buy a home in the coming year. Saving every dollar, we can.

Sometimes I do just want to quit trying or pushing myself. I just get tired of it all. Of all the obstacles, the fails and trails I'm put through that I was once able to do. I know it's my depression kicking in. I now have depression because of the AVM. I hate it but I have to deal with it. If I'm sad I think of a good ole memory to lift me up. I mostly think of my Papa who is watching over me now. I think of our talks and his home-made chocolate syrup! How sweet and yummy it was. I smile instantly no matter of I have eyes full of tears. I hear his voice in my head telling me to "cowgirl up!" He is and will always be my, " cowboy angel!" When it's not quite time for me to take my depression medicine I just think of him and that is a good dose. Does me good!

The journey I have had, and that I am still travelling, is a long road. I realize I may have had the AVM but it's also affected my family. It is said that those who have AVM's are born with them, and it's just like a time bomb, you don't know when it will go off. Mine just happened to be in the middle of night.

AVM/Aneurysms are hereditary, so we are getting our daughters checked. This is a life changing event for sure. I had to learn to walk again. I'm still wobbly, and I will always be, and I will always have a cane. Balance issues, my taste buds, endurance, sleepiness, headaches I pay attention to them all now, because I know it can happen again.

On a touchy subject, I am going to address how I feel about adult entertainers. I wasn't always comfortable with my body. I didn't even have rhythm. I wasn't ashamed of my looks just not happy. How did I start? A friend and I went to armature night and after one round on all the stages, that was seven dances total, I was way over two-hundred dollars. Having that money in my hand, in such a short amount of time just dancing, which I did enjoy, made my choice very easy. Still I had no rhythm, although other people seemed to think I did.

Knowing I had no rhythm I had to do something. I watched the others and I picked out the one I wanted to go to and ask for help. She took me under her wing and taught me daily until I learned and it became natural to me.

There are some girls out there who take advantage of this environment meaning they act like they are entertainers but really they proposition the men. I don't and never have liked these women. You learn fast who they are.

You have your bad experiences along with the good. I think if you put mine on a scale they may equal out the same. I've had drug dealers ask me for drugs even ask if they could pay me in drugs. I would simply say "You have the wrong girl".

Some good experience I was actually paid by a wonderful couple to teach the wife to dance for her husband. He gave me the money said he would be back later to get his wife.

These moments seeing the wife so happy she was able to make her husband the night he will remember was just enough to make me smile and say " I did that".

Over the years you bond with some girls and soon y'all coincident one another family. Always going to one another's birthdays even the kid's birthdays. Celebrate your birthday at work. Yes, dancing was work.

One of the more positive benefits from dancing was that I was able to gain a better self-esteem over there years! I was very proud of the way I looked and danced. When my name was called to stage, the whole club would stop what they were doing and watch. From a girl with no rhythm to a woman with all the moves! I was that one everyone knew and wanted to watch! I didn't care about the money I just loved to put on a great show!

The music you choose has to be your style or you just won't look or do good. I danced to a variety. From blue grass, to hard rock then some classics. It's mostly whatever I was feeling that day or whatever the DJ or boss was itching to hear.

I have met some celebrities. I can tell you fame had gotten to them. They treated you different that's for sure. Some demanded attention while others were very laid back and just wanted company. You get the vibe then decide if it's your cup of tea or not. I have walked away from one celebrity and past on the money. I believe in Karma still today!

That celebrity you can say was a one hit wonder singer. I'm so glad I didn't stay and I don't care who you are~ you show respect to woman! All the sweaty dollar bills I was tipped went to my family's expenses! All I'm saying is it doesn't matter if you're the best looking or the girl with no rhythm in the club, you're going to make money. When you leave to go home every girl walks out of that club feeling heart ache, feeling ashamed cause of how they are seen by the world it society. When you go into a club and you see that random girl you don't know her road or story. But know she has one, they all do.

As far as I am aware of I was living in great health and then one day with no warning this AVM came and took away so much. Things like AVMs can bring out the best in people that survive them. I have changed from the person I was prior to my AVM to the person I am now. I was not so sympathetic to others as to their feelings, don't get me wrong I wasn't mean. I just wasn't as nice and sympathetic as I am today. I care so much about people around the world even our pets. I cry often when I see a show or a commercial about the pain or whatever it maybe that they are going through. I wish them all happiness and the feel of joy.

I wish someone had told me anything about AVM's or Aneurysms. I wasn't aware of anything. It was a time bomb in my head just waiting to go off with no warning to me. I hope whoever reads my story of my path or road may help a little. I really hope it brings a little awareness out into the world.

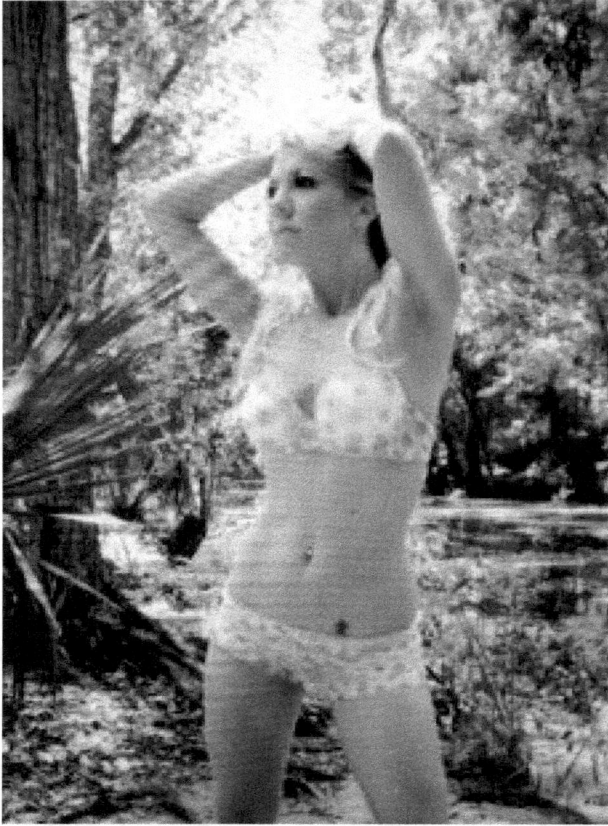

CHAPTER SIX

What I wish I had known…..

Some things I wish I was told:

When the AVM decided to go off I would have the worse headache of my life. I thought I was in a crash. I literally was telling my husband to check in the other people who was in the crash. I wasn't worried about my own life at the time.

You lose your balance when you try to walk. I was walking like I was drunk.

You black out and may not remember anything that is going on at that moment.

Catheters are embarrassing. Having to somehow hide it when it's bigger than the bag your trying to hide it in, and tie it on the walker.

Walkers are not pretty in decorations. They put blue tennis balls on the bottom of my walker so it would slide easier.

You cannot sleep in the hospital. Between the cords wrapping around you constantly and the nurses walking in all the time.

They will shave your hair if they need too. This today has scared me. I love my hair.

They will poke you every day with needles. Always needing

something or giving you something. It hurt. I bruised.

These things I really wish someone would have shared with me what to expect.

I have spent some time learning and using a walker, and I was not happy about it at all. It wasn't pretty, matter of fact, it was a plain silver color and they put blue tennis balls on the front legs for it to slide/ move easy for me. If you want, you can buy any color tennis balls to put on the front legs to add some color to the walker. I have seen some people use those bright neon green ones also yellow. After that plain silver walker I went to a walker that had a bucket type thing where you could turn around and sit on it if you needed too. That thing looked even worse than the other walker. Because of this I have thought of a cool hip walker design. If I had money I sure would put a Patton on my idea. Someone needs to do something, the world needs cute, hip walkers for young people. This may help some by them not being embarrassed to be using one. The current ones just look old and not something young people should be using.

We like that funky stuff! Someone definitely needs to design a new walker. Maybe one day I can do my idea that would be really awesome! I do not have a "therapy" dog. Although My family does own a blue nose pit bull, which I consider my "therapy dog." I am thinking about registering her as one because she has helped me emotionally and still does on a daily basis. Her name is Harley. She is my daily dose of happiness (other than coffee) since I'm home alone during the day. Everyone is either at school or work.

I am now at home doing what I can around the house. During the minutes that I don't have anything to do, I play with my dog Harley. She brings me her toy she wants to play with, I say to her " let's do therapy." This means I use only my left hand to hold the toy she chose to play with. We play tug a war, I play with my arm that is very weak from my AVM. She understands this somehow. She gives and takes the right amount to where I use my strength in my arm. This helps me build my muscle back. We play till one if us gives in and let's go of the toy. It is fun to both of us.

Harley is a gift. It really is the other way around I believe. She is spoiled. Sleeps in the middle of Alex and I, also with Sydnee. She steels the covers and snores like a human.

Tending to her is my therapy. I kennel her up when we go somewhere if she doesn't come with us. We take her to Galveston with us. She knows the words " load up." She knows when we go to get a drink she gets her own. She takes showers. She is a very spoiled but loving dog to my family.

I'm blessed to having her in my life. Emotionally she is the one I go to during the day. She can look at me and I can just talk and vent away, of course I know she is a dog and can't answer. But that doesn't matter to me, she listens and loves on me every day. She is my therapy.

One thing that I want to say, this is my opinion. When you have problems, problems with learning, problems with memory or problems with speech, you are very self-conscious. While those you love may not be judging you, you even judge yourself. It is hard not to think that other's do not notice your struggles when you yourself do. I know that at times I am my toughest critic, Harley has never judged me. Harley loves me and smiles when I am happy, and gives me wet puppy loves when I am not. Harley is the one and only I cannot worry about anything with. I really recommend a companion pet for all of those who need one.

CHAPTER SEVEN

My Journal and Personal Thoughts

A journal is a private and personal way to record your thoughts. I have found it therapeutic. I debated with myself to share this. I have decided to share because if there is one person reading this book who has gone through what I have, I want you to know- you are not alone in this. We share the same frustrations, challenges, thoughts. We are family and we are on this crazy journey together. The other reason I decided to add these journal entries is this. If one mother or father of a AVM/Aneurysm or brain injury victim is reading this, searching for understanding, I hope this helps. This is a real struggle and you are not alone, none of us are alone in this.

My journal entry's during my therapy:

January 6,2014
There are so many problems and situations when you get effected by an AVM. Your self-esteem lowers, your looks change, people treat you different, you lose confidence, some people think different about you maybe.

I want to walk around the Harry Potter world and show the world how having my Avm has affected me and you can survive afterwards! There is still hope! By the looks of it I may not experience this trip but in the long run it doesn't matter! I am HERE! I walked around looking at Christmas lights and it was exhausting but I *did it*! I don't care who looked at me thinking, *what happened to her*? I am just so happy I could do it! My self-esteem is gaining!

January 6, 2014

Here is some insight into how I am making a recovery back to "my normal self" that people still marvel at today. I tell myself to: Believe in myself. Don't give up. Do it for yourself. Be you. Dream big!

January 7, 2014

Another dividing line that separates the survivors from the onlookers is the social aspects of life. The survivors realize that they should spend less time worrying about work and the small things and spending more time with their friends and family. When the survivors spend time with their family they think of it as extra time for that it's time they might not have had, yet for the people who are just onlookers their time spent with the survivors is completely different.

When the onlookers spend time with survivors they cannot stop thinking about all the pain and trouble the survivor had to go through. All they can focus on is the bad not the good. The onlookers are always feeling this sense of sorrow when they should be feeling appreciative because they are able to spend more time with someone they almost lost.

January 7, 2014

A brain aneurysm is a major-medical problem that people die from every year, usually because they were not aware of the signs and symptoms. For the ones who are aware and lucky enough to survive face many day-to-day problems. These problems range anywhere from medical problems to problems with how they are treated by outsiders who are not aware of what they are going through. Due to this, there is a major dividing line between the survivors of an aneurysm and the people just observing the survivors.

January 7,2014

This is my second day of looking into my new me. Some patients are able to care for themselves after a short period of recovery. It is important to keep in mind that each of us is unique and recovery times vary.

This journey can be made easier with support from healthcare, family and friends, strength and courage to survive. Everyone thinks they are helping but they're not. I wish they knew.

January 13,2014

After the worst was over, my slow recovery began. I don't know how long I was in the hospital. I cried almost every day; the feeling of helplessness was awful. For the first weeks, I couldn't stand so I lost all muscle definition. For the first few weeks after that it felt like my body had forgotten how to walk and I was dizzy all the time and very heavy headed.

January 13,2014

But as the weeks passed, I realized I could only keep getting better. I still have down days, I still cry over nothing and I'll forever be asking "Why?", but then I remember that months ago I was almost dead, and today I'm almost back to normal. I still get tired easily and don't sleep well, which are common symptoms of a brain trauma injury.

January 14, 2014

By sharing our information with others, in lessening another's pain, we still can experience gain. In many ways, we are now a new person old dreams must somehow be put to rest. How do we figure out what is realistic? Will we know the right path to follow? We have felt a beginning and also an end. We must somehow say good-bye to the old. It is frightening to find a new beginning, never knowing if we can possibly succeed. We must stop wasting time and move forward, we have to let go of "what has been" before.

January 29,2014
I believe I sat my goal high but I added all the expenses into it, seems difficult but not impossible. You don't want the bar so high that you'll never reach it, but you want to keep it high enough that you'll push your effort to get there. I've tried. I pushed. Picture yourself doing what it takes to succeed, and you will soon find yourself believing that you can. And the best part, is that your absolutely right. I may not be going to universal studios to show everyone I'm still here and my esteem is gaining but that doesn't bring me down! I'm here, I'm stronger, I'm alive! I am a survivor! Thank you all who have donated and supported me on this goal. I love and adore you all!

September 3,2014
You don't necessary see the physical disabilities with brain aneurysm patients, and their families sometimes get frustrated with them because while they may look like they are back to normal, they're not acting normal. Then the survivors get upset because nobody understands their situation and they have nobody to talk to about it. When an aneurysm does rupture, the foundation says, about 15 percent of the victims die before even reaching a hospital.

Physical therapy began almost at once as it is believed that timing is everything in teaching our bodies to respond to our new mind, my new mind. Once settled in the rehab center, I began a vigorous daily schedule of physical, occupational, speech and cognitive therapies. I would have to relearn the most tasks that we all take for granted, such as bathing, dressing, walking, and eating. It all came back to me! I even had to relearn the process of swallowing liquids because I only liked to swallow on one side. I was taken very good care of by both men and women and of course family and friends helped in any way they could. My nurses were amazing although some were not so. My family made sure those didn't come back. Through time and hard work, I continued to improve daily, though my left side was slow to recover. I graduated from a wheel chair to a walker. This of course was over many weeks of therapy, hard work and my own determination.

My walker became active in my therapeutic rehabilitation and family passed along my triumphs to both other family members and friends. No one let me rest or escaped my scheduled therapy sessions. I had therapy in the hospital known as in- patient. I now see it as a good thing, but at the time I found everything and most everybody to be an intrusion. I wanted to be left alone, however no one would let me be. Good thing - they all had a lot to do with my recovery. I had been a healthy 5'2 110 pound 36-year-old, who neither drank alcohol nor smoked. I was an active model. Just days before this I had a photo shoot!

Unfortunately, all these preventative measures cannot overcome what we are born with, but they have been acknowledged as playing a big part in my subsequent survival and recovery. The hospital called me " the miracle" people who wasn't even family or a friend came into the room just to see " the miracle". This was odd at times but I was very happy. The hospital also knew I was a model. My wonderful family put pictures of my last shoot up on the wall behind my bed so everyone could see. Now, I am learning to live my life as an independent confident woman. With The constructive support and encouragement of family, friends and a dedicated therapy staff, I am becoming physically and emotionally stronger each day.

Prior to my bleed, I worked as a tireless perfectionist. I loved my work, my coworkers and boss's. I enjoyed being a woman and was even preoccupied, in looking my best. I now keep my hair short and am pleased with the look. Makeup has become a rare activity. I still very much enjoy being a woman, now just a natural woman. I am alive and again looking forward to enjoying life each day, at the highest possible level. I want everyone to be aware of how important headaches or migraines are. I don't mess around now and just take an Advil or 2, if I scale it above my normal rate we go ahead to the place I can't stand. The ER. Someday I may surprise everyone and do a shoot just for the hell of it. I would love to be an advocate for aneurysm model survivors if there was a such thing.

September 2014

What is an AVM you ask? It stands for an arteriovenous malformation and is a mass of incorrectly formed blood vessels that shaped in my brain before I was born. It is rare and is almost never identified before one of these "bad" blood vessels break, causing a hemorrhage in the brain and usually death or severe physical or mental handicaps. I was one of the "lucky ones" I survived. you know how I did it? Well with people praying for me, my family by my side encouraging me day and night, and my friends visiting me in the hospital. They had me in therapy from 8 o'clock every weekday morning until four or four-thirty in the afternoon. It was immensely tiring and a lot of hard work, but they got me from a wheelchair, to a walker.

The night that I had that bleed, I had what I now call a "totally awesome near death experience." I saw my grandma and uncle who had passed away. While in the hospital my uncle and grandma would come into my room and mess with the machine (I'm guessing the IV machine) and make the noises go off. Then the nurses would come in. My grandma would put her finger to her mouth and say "shah" so I didn't say anything I just let the nurses do their thing. When I became better enough to talk about things I told that to my family. And they told me the machines really went off and the nurses came in often to fix the noise. I think my uncle was making those noises go off so the nurses would go in. Also, my grandma would hold my hand and sing the song she always sung to me when she wanted. I'll never forget that song and that moment. It was a great near death experience I hope that doesn't sound bad.

Going through a "totally spiritual experience" like that changed my life. Back in my "rebellious teen" days, I used to not be what they call churchy. I'm still not but I do go to church now. I do believe. I believe in miracles. But now that

I've had this bleed and spiritual experience behind me, my outlook has been altered. My whole attitude towards life has really started to change since then. My whole attitude towards life has really started to change since then too. Now, instead of feeling sorry for myself, I've decided that there must be some reason for my survival. That life is to be lived and enjoyed no matter how long or short it is. That anyone can make a difference no matter who they are.

September 3,2014

I just want people to know that no matter how bad you think things are, and no matter how black the hole you seem to be in is, there is a light at the end, things do get better, you just need to remain positive in any way that you can, and know that you can get through it, and that on the other side things are so much better! I just wish I could hurry and get to that other side.

September 17,2014

Everyone's story and intention is different. You can't let someone else's interpretation of your dreams define who you are and how you feel about it. I've learned what's important to me is "not to be defined by my old work, but by the person I am.

This aneurysm has really taken a toll on me and my thoughts, also how I am now.

I know firsthand that having success alone, is not going to fill you up. Looking back, I recall a few career highlights (model gigs) that are wonderful to have had the experience of, but at the end of the day, weren't my happiest stages in life. I did learn! You have to put yourself out there and take risks. Sink or swim. You have to give things a try. Experience and discover the growth within yourself that challenges in life gives you. appreciate that gift that's only given through times of struggle and hardship. I'm finding new things out that I didn't know I would enjoy! I look forward to becoming 100% recovered so I can experience more! I have gone on and on so I'll let you go! I just wanted to let you yes YOU know no matter what the challenge Is for you, don't give up!

I haven't! Also, no matter what they say (random people) words hurt yes but don't let them bring you down. STAY YOU, STAY STRONG!

September 3,2014
You don't necessary see the physical disabilities with brain aneurysm patients, and their families sometimes get frustrated with them because while they may look like they are back to normal, they're not acting normal. Then the survivors get upset because nobody understands their situation and they have nobody to talk to about it. I totally can relate to this. When an aneurysm does rupture, the foundation says, about 15 percent of the victims die before reaching a hospital. They thought I was over dosing.

November 14, 2014
I am preparing for something very important in my life, and I am asking for your moral, financial, and emotional support. Why is this important to me? Everyone knows my survival story but doesn't fully know what I have gone through. It is a very long tough journey I admit. I want to build my endurance up to where I can stand and walk longer. I get very faintish feeling if I stand or walk for period of time that is one way this has affected me.

Many people say I'm their inspiration and although I am so thankful for that I feel I do not deserve to be. I just want to acknowledge that anyone can go through this horrible tragedy. I wish this upon NOONE.

My aneurysm was very rare, called an AVM. For those who don't know what this is, it's aka arteriovenous malformation. I was born with it. It was just time that no one could change. It was my AVM's time to explode in my brain. AVM is an abnormal connection between arteries and veins. An AVM is usually congenital, meaning it dates to birth. An AVM can develop anywhere in your body but occurs most often in the brain or spine. A brain AVM, which appears as a tangle of abnormal arteries and veins, can occur in any part of your brain. The cause isn't clear. You may not know you have a brain AVM until you experience symptoms, such as headaches or a seizure. In serious cases, the blood vessels rupture, causing bleeding in the brain (hemorrhage). Once diagnosed, a brain AVM can cause death.

I was care-flighted and had the best surgeons in Houston. I'm lucky to be here. While at the hospital there were four others that were experiencing an aneurysm. They did not make it. After word got around that I made it I became known as the miracle girl. I don't remember much about the early stages of my stay at the ER but I was put in ICU. I believe I stayed awhile. My family stayed and slept on the floor. I feel bad I know that horrible hard cold floor was not comfortable. The nurses kept me very and I do mean very drugged up. I almost died because I was being over drugged. My family is who figured that out and saved my life by telling the nurses and doctors to stop some meds. My family took great care of me!

I don't remember much of what happened like I said and if my family didn't do a daily journal about what happened daily I would have never known. By reading the journal they made I learned that my cousin flew in from Indiana to see me, my childhood best friend and still is drove from our home town, that's far, all my family and some friends came. All of them took time to write in the journal.

They were all told it would be their last time to see me. That's so sad. My mom held my hand and I was unconscious she told me to move my hand if I could hear her. I did. That's when everyone found out I'm a survivor! This girl is a miracle. I have never wanted to share pictures that family took while I was in the hospital because I guess I'm ashamed of them. I guess because I didn't take care of my headaches I had before.

This has impacted my life a lot. Everything is harder for me to do now. Things you take for granted. Stepping on stairs, making a peanut butter and jelly sandwich, tying your shoes. Those are just some. My speech is very different now. I get tired just from talking. My balance is messed up. I have graduated from speech and will graduate from my physical therapy soon. I continue to work daily on my progress even though I'm graduated from speech. I plan on continuing on getting better on my physical therapy as well. I plan on reaching 100% or close.

My self-esteem is very low now cause of this. I'm working on that and by me attending this very populated park will help not only my esteem but also my therapy! Me being seen by others is a very big deal to me I know it's weird but maybe because I was a model. Allowing others to see me will show others that, I am that miracle girl! I am the girl that survived!

I am going to share some of the things I wrote along my journey. I am still writing; I write every day. These are just some of my writings when I first started writing my memories. Before I let you go I want you to know it's very important to me to go to universal studios the Harry Potter park and walk and take pictures like I used to do. Most important share those pictures with you all because you are the reason I'm here today!

November 14,2014
Now, this to me is normal and I know I need to slow down and not do too many things at once but explaining this to my family is a different story. I don't know if they can't accept me for who I am now or they refuse to believe that I am not exactly the same person but it makes me sad. One of the things I am realizing that I need with this aneurysm is not just the good health, but a good heart. I find myself needing patience for myself and others - especially others. I need forgiveness for those who do not understand what an aneurysm is, let alone how one is fixed. I need patience and

understanding so that I can educate them with time and example. And then forgiveness again when it doesn't always work.

June 26th 2013 was a bad night for my family. That is the night I developed the worst headache of my life. That's when my story of my aneurysm starts. The ambulance medics thought I overdosed. The ER figured out I was having an aneurysm and care flighted me to a hospital that knew how to help me. The next two weeks were spent hooked up to the machines and drips. I would throw up everything. The staff were fabulous but it was my family that kept me sane. Seeing them at visiting time was like cool water on a hot day.

I was taken from ICU to the rehab hospital, the brain aneurysm was not stopping me! I did every exercise, every task 3 or 4 times more than the times I was asked to! I wanted to get back home to my life so bad. My family and home town friend was in the waiting room praying I'm sure. after my surgery and they were told to go home and rest, my family slept on the floor in my room. Others left but came back every day. They wouldn't leave my side. I'm so sorry I know that floor is uncomfortable and cold. They kept a journal that they all took turns writing in daily. Most wrote about what I did that day or how they felt.

I remember being so tired of chocolate pudding. I'm sure the taste of it now will make me want to throw up. I couldn't swallow big pills so they crushed them and mixed them into chocolate pudding. Learning how to eat was a good thing! Rehab was grueling, but necessary. I have never worked so hard in my life. Just daily rituals came hard. Nurses I thanked so much. I hated being poked by needles every day. They hurt but I tried to not show the pain.

November 23,2014
Everyone asks how I'm feeling all the time. I tell them "I'm good. I feel like my body is back to normal." My physical body feels fine. My emotional, mental, and spiritual body has

been to hell and back. I survived a very large rupture. Nothing can stop me. I feel like God has so much purpose for me on earth. I'm superwoman.

I feel like my life is still worth living somehow. I honestly can't tell you why. When I look at everything I've been through, everything I've lost, I feel like there is just not much left. Deep down I feel like I still have a good life, it's just not how I wanted it to be. It's something I can't really explain.

There's just so many emotions involved with having an AVM. It's so hard to explain to people, especially because I appear normal on the outside now. It's hard to explain to people that some days I just have to avoid certain situations because my emotions get out of control and I get really physically sick. I wish people would just tell me it's ok to be sad or mad or disappointed or confused. I wish people could accept my emotions. I feel like so many people mean well by telling me to "Look on the bright side" and "Be thankful you're alive", but it makes me so ashamed of my true feelings sometimes. I want someone to listen to me without interrupting with a thousand suggestions about how to be happy. I fear becoming emotionally numb.

November 23,2014
I feel angry. So so angry. Why did this happen to me? Why am I 37 years old and having to learn how to walk again? Why can't I fold clothes right? Why can't I stand for a while? Why does everyone question my every action? I feel so angry that I am not independent.

November 24,2014
I'm so tired of being tired. My mind is constantly racing. My body is constantly tense. I relax for a couple of days but then I just lose it again. Dealing with everything is just so exhausting. I wish I could just sleep all day.

November 30,2014
There will be challenges to face and changes to make in your life, and it is up to you to accept them. Constantly keep yourself headed in the right direction for you not anyone

else. It may not be easy at times, but in those times of struggle you will find a stronger sense of who you are, so when the days come that are filled with frustration and unexpected responsibilities, remember to believe in yourself and all you want your life to be, because the challenges and changes will only help you to find the goals that you know are meant to come true for you. Keep believing in yourself. +++

May 20,2015

I had my time in the spot light. Now it's time for someone else to shine. It saddens me but it's true.

July 31,2015

Reality is, I have had to come to terms with many broken dreams. I have to depend on others, something I would have never dreamed of. Time has taught me to let go, the broken dreams have taught me humility. Now time is spent planning a new future, developing new dreams and goals. I am never sure if dreams will come true, but hope is a gift that I give myself.

The disappointment is always there just under the surface, of what could have been. This year has not taken away the wounds, it has just taught me to deal with them. The internal struggle every day to do the things that were once so easy makes me sad. But then I look around me and I know that it could be much worse, and I feel thankful. I still believe broken dreams can be mended, and I choose to spend my energy there.

Reality. Can I get a 'roll eye'? Seriously. What is Reality? We all have our own idea or concept of what realm of reality we live in. Some of us live in our perfect perception of it, while others of us struggle always feeling as though we are so small and everything is about to come crashing down anytime.

My reality has changed. I always believed that if you tried hard and focused you can accomplish anything you set out too. That is no longer true. I no longer have the energy, I have headaches, I avoid large crowds, and on and on and on. I am not the same person.

My reality? The only certainty is the sun will set and the sun will raise. I died, I learn a little bit about the new me every day.

August 28,2015
Our family is especially appreciative of the many prayers, words of encouragement and support we've received from family and friends. My improvement is made each day and shows. "I am thankful to God for my survival and for his patience with my continuous straying and complaining, yet he has never given up, and I find that my faith continues to increase! many have asked me how I am doing. How very grateful I am for the love and concern expressed by everyone. I have had a number of individuals tell me that they wanted to share my journey with other aneurysm patients who are currently going through their own journeys. I will never be able to express my deepest gratitude to all of you who have prayed for me and encouraged me with emails, texts, visits, and notes of encouragement. Please know that I am grateful beyond words for your love. Please continue! I can and will do this!

September 18,2015
Today I wrote as a guest on one of my high school teachers blog. This is what I wrote.

Don't let anyone take away your shine. Dream big, never give up! Stay strong, keep up the good work and keep on keeping on. Those are just a few things that you hear that may keep you going. Well know this, your never alone, your dreams can become reality, and you are someone special. Everyone has bad days and everyone has a dream. You just need to decide if you're that type of person who will strive to make that dream come true or just "let it go." No matter your situation, reach for the stars! Do not give up hope! Look around, you may see a random feather or a penny! There is always good luck around. Feathers are a sign of angels! So, that one feather you saw beside you, maybe your angel! See you're not ever alone!

CPR Helps Mostek Employees Save Child

Wendy Launius is spending this Christmas season at home. Maybe that's not so unusual for an 18-month-old infant, but were it not for Mostek Corp. employees Jim Gaspard and Silvia Waters the Launius and Rains household at 2017 North Broadway in Carrollton might not have much to celebrate this year.

Gaspard, who works as a program manager for trade shows in the advertising department, and Mrs. Waters, who is a registered nurse and heads the Mostek clinic, are credited with saving Wendy's life during a recent incident at the Mostek facility on Crosby Road.

Heroes and heroines are hard to find, so when the Carrollton City Council discovers worthy candidates it honors them with special recognition. Gaspard and Mrs. Waters were honored during the Dec. 18 city council meeting with a certificate of special commendation for service to the community.

When Wendy's mother came to Mostek to apply for a job in November, she left her baby with Patricia Rains, her mother, in a parked car near Mostek's employment center.

Mrs. Rains noticed that Wendy's breathing suddenly changed and that she started staring vacantly. Mrs. Rains took the baby in her arms screaming for someone to call an ambulance as she approached Gaspard, who was working in the advertising loading dock area.

Gaspard, who has had previous emergency training as a Navy medic, acted quickly; he grabbed Wendy from her grandmother's arms while shouting for someone to call the Mostek Clinic.

Meanwhile, Wendy stopped breathing. As Gaspard ran through the foyer of the employment center with Mrs. Rains behind, Wendy's mother, Debbie Launius, joined the race. The trio left a trail of footprints in the wet concrete of the parking lot.

When they reached the clinic, Mrs. Waters performed CPR to get the baby breathing again. It worked. Later Wendy was taken to Parkland Memorial Hospital where a series of tests was performed to discover why she went into convulsion. After a week of tests, doctors decided that a low blood sugar level resulting from a case of flu caused her convulsion.

Both Gaspard and Mrs. Waters shy away from any publicity about saving Wendy's life. Gaspard said: "I was just scared. So I started running."

Mrs. Waters said, "When that baby started breathing again that was all the reward I needed."

Both Gaspard and Mrs. Waters stressed the importance of learning CPR and enrolling in refresher courses to keep up-to-date on the latest advances in medical treatment.

Mrs. Launius, Wendy

Gaspard, Waters

June 26th will be the 2-year anniversary of my AVM. We've all heard that old saying about a picture being worth a thousand words. But looks can be quit deceiving. A face smiling back at you as you look at a picture tells you so little. A little over 2 years ago, on a day like today, the old Wendy died.

I was woken up by a headache unlike any before around 1am on that fateful day in June. I write now, to create a record of this journey, one that I hope to look back on with delight as I see progress. During my hospital stay my family and friends kept a daily journal of their thoughts and also my daily happenings. I look at this often reading what all happened to me and how they felt.

Many of my new friends are in the same AVM/aneurysm group on Facebook that I am in. I open my heart and soul to let others know that they are not alone, that others share in their challenges and truly understand. And I write so that I can try to better understand my own new life. My goal today is to offer a bit of a picture as to what my daily life is like as I start year three of life since my accident. An AVM or aneurysm is like a shadow on a sunny day. It follows you everywhere you go. No matter how fast you run, no matter how high you jump, there is no escaping your shadow.

My AVM is always there. Sure, there are moments that I don't think about it. Like that shadow, you know it's there. Just look down and you'll always see it. But it never goes away. Ever. AVM/Aneurysms are often called a hidden disability. Most who may see a picture of me and Alex would think we look like a couple of fun people out living life. That's true, but there is so much more. Don't let anyone kid you. Brain aneurysms effect everyone involved. Wives, husbands, mothers, fathers, sisters, children, aunts, uncles, cousins the list goes on. All are impacted by an AVM/Aneurysm.

About a year of therapy did not eliminate the challenges I face now. I can no longer tolerate crowds for any length of time, the noise bothers me, my balance is horrible, I'm with a cane at this young age. It's one of those odd things of a head trauma that is difficult to even begin to explain. It hurts my feelings to even try to explain. Survivors know. If you see me somewhere, and I do nothing more than smile and say hello, you would never know what life is like behind the smile. But I do.

It's one of those frustrations I try not to even think about, as nothing can be done about it. But it's not all tears. Though all of this, I have been met some of the most inspirational people I have ever met... my fellow survivors in our online groups– people whose life make mine look like a cake walk. I have met caring therapist who are truly compassionate in their care. I've had complete strangers reach out to me with kindness after they hear my story. I'm told I'm an inspiration to many and I can't tell you how much that means to me! The Bigger Picture is now clearer to me.

At times, I look around and "see" with my eyes in a way I

never knew possible. And the smaller things in life have taken on new meaning. I find myself wrapping my arms around Alex several times a day. Not needing any type of reassurance, I find simple pleasure in just holding him.

The ocean stops me dead in my tracks, it's power I have so much respect and admiration for. My near death has slowed my pace, and that is good thing. Time has already shown that my experience as a survivor makes me uniquely qualified to help other survivors. I "get it" from an insider's perspective and I have had real world experience through rebuilding my life.

I feel a deep sense of responsibility to use the voice that I have. In helping others, I have found a peace. And for that, I am profoundly grateful. I'm a survivor! Going on 2 years now!

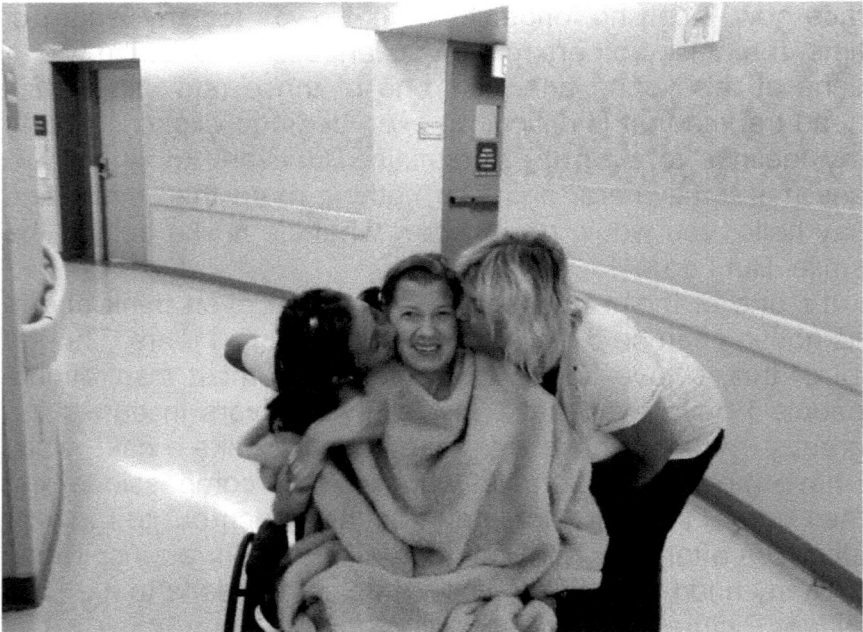

THE HOSPITAL JOURNAL:

Going forward, I try to help other survivors and their families. Dealing with any type of brain trauma is difficult for all involved. After careful consideration, I decided to include my family's person journal they took while I was in the hospital. It was a day to day struggle. I am including this in the book, not because it is good reading, it is not. I am including it for those who need hope. Keep in mind, the doctors had no idea if I was ever going to open my eyes. They had no idea if I would ever talk, know my name, or ever walk again. My family was at the ultimate low when this was written. Also, keep in mind, we never thought I would write this book either.

Day 1
Noon- 12 Alex/Sydnee(daughter)/ Debbie(mom)/Meagan(sister)- Wendy cough Sydnee took picture
1:00-Alex/Debbie/Traci(aunt)- feet fixed straight; hands loose; one breathe per 4 seconds
2:00-Alex/Alyssa
3:00- Alex- nurse sucking chest out Wendy tears fall down cheek, spit up
4:00-5:00- Wendy is resting. Debbie, Meagan,Sydnee,Alex/, Alyssa/Tyler(cousin) go eat at Denny's
6:00 Katrina (cat) misses you
7:00 going to do another catscan to make sure still okay- looks really good
8:00- 6-8 shift change no visitors
8:15- Adrian(step dad)/ Ty/ Sherry(Step sister) in Houston
9:00-Debbie with Wendy- she lifted her arm to push nurse away, blinking
10:00- Ty/ Adrian/Sherry-here

11:00- Debbie/Adrian/ Sherry/ Ty/Traci- moving around, moving legs, moving right/ left leg on command, Dr. Asked her to move her right thumb up and she did it

Thursday
June 27,2013
12:00-4:00am- Adrian/Meagan/Sherry/Sydnee -hotel
Ty/Traci/Tyler-visit: Alyssa-with neighbor for school Debbie/Alex- stay with Wendy. She will probably have a drain tube the rest of her life/ small hidden behind ear- if feels pressure she can push to release pressure
5:00-11:00 doctors are excited and shocked " miracle"
She crossed legs she is comfortable Pictures angiogram-line through leg release dye, see veins, Moved around

Day 2
Dr. asked her to help slide over to bed
12:00- angiogram and pictures look awesome Cyndi(childhood best friend)
1:00-2:00 She is resting, Debbie/Adrian/ Meagan/Sherry/ Sydnee/Alyssa/Ty/Tyler/Cyndi-go eat ; Traci -waiting room
3:00- Debbie/Adrian/ Sydnee/ Alyssa/ Ty/Tyler- went to go rest a little Meagan/Cyndi/Sherry/ Alex- stayed
4:00 Meagan/Cyndi told you, you were moving back home and you shook your head " yes"!
5:00- Nurse Shannon told you we are having a big party with all your friends cause you're a miracle child... You gave him a huge thumbs up.
6:00 no visitations, it's killing us we can't come in and see you.
7:00- nurse says your doing great and opening your eyes frequently
8:00- making movements like hurting. Alex asked where you hurt you moved arm in a circle motion as to you hurt all over.
9:00 they are talking about taking tube out.
10:00- fever 101, neighbor family came to visit you. Eyes looking a little off
11:00- Valerie (Sherry's daughter, Wendy's step niece) put your picture on her Facebook photo and several others did

too. Putting nutrition through your tube., breathing good, crossing legs

Friday June 28,2013
CEO of the hospital talked to Alex happy about your progress

12:00 midnight- Alex/Sherry/Cyndi/Traci- stayed all night

1:00- turn down sedation- asked her to lift legs, arms, wiggle toes, 100 temperature

2:00- 100.4 temperature, digesting everything!

3:00- wakes to louder voice(almost never happens)!

4:00-eyes look good, looked at Alex! Everyone excited at the hospital how well she's doing.

5:00- raise left hand, wants to pull tube out but stops when told to stop.

6:00- morning cough, cross legs

7/8:00-Alex rubbing foot- she did her hands side to side as to stop rubbing them.

9:00-we all decided to do a Wendy support ribbon bracelet (pink with crosses)

9:27pm- Wendy ate all her dinner. She had cream of chicken soup and chocolate pudding. She ate all of it. Even the pudding and she hates chocolate pudding. She said she wanted a shake the pudding was nasty.

Day 3
12noon-

2:00pm- they took out breathing tube.

3:00- first question asked after tube out " what is your name?" You answered " Wendy!"

4:00- now you can talk to all of us, love hearing your voice. Your asking everyone where their pink ribbon

was as you point at yours in your hair. That made you very happy seeing us where the ribbons.

5:00- dr gave you mess by mouth, you saw how much they wanted to give you, you said," oh shit!"

 7-11:00- no entry

 * all day long we had a lady bug sit on one of the chairs with us. We all thought it was strange, but we will take all the

good luck!

Day 4 June 29,2013

12:00- occupational therapist came in, she did great. Did everything you were asked to do. It was kind of hard for you to hold your head u, but you did it. Then they brought you the walker and you reached for it ready to go. You were able to stand by yourself and look up at me(Traci) and Cyndi, you did so amazing. When you laid back down I was leaving, I let you know and you looked at me and you said," I love you so much", best thing ever!

12:00 lunch came, you had chicken purée and purée peas and carrots, you didn't like it at all. You had sweet tea to drink. Not much tasted good to you.

5:00pm- doing more therapy, worked with legs, arms and eyes. You did everything perfect.

6:00- Aaron(cousin) was able to call you and talk to you.

8:00- went into visit you and you made the girls and I laugh so hard! You were cracking jokes and evil eying me. I tried to wipe your mouth with a tissue, the look you shot at me made me laugh so hard my belly hurt. Then you making that " Elvis lip" Too funny.

Sunday June 30,2013

12:00 midnight- you kept wanting to go home and looking for your phone. Kept trying to get up and pulling at catheter.

1:00am- continued wanting to get up and go home.

2-3 same

4:00- went for ct scan came back and complained of head hurting. Nurse gave you pain medicine 5:00- finally you went to sleep

6-7:00- sleep

8:00am- Shannon came in and adjusted your drip machine. Winging you from drip line, cleaned and replaced drip line fluid bag.

9:00- breakfast came 1 scrambled egg and cream of wheat, ate 3 spoon dulls of egg and 2 of cream of wheat.

10:00- Dr. Shih (neurology surgeon) came and evaluated

you. Said you was doing good. Therapy came only worked with you for a few minutes, you started to complain about head hurting. Nurse gave you pain medicine.

July 4,2013
Alex/Sydnee/Alyssa/Debbie /Meagan-at hospital all week: You called fireworks ," boom booms."

July 6,2013
Took tube out of head, good therapy, good smiles- kisses
Out of Icu into room Sydnee/Alex/Debbie- stay all week

This is where the entries ended. I can only imagine what my family and friends were going through during this time. I do not know why they decided to keep a journal. I am very happy they did. I do not remember any of this. Looking back, this helped me to understand. For that, I am grateful.

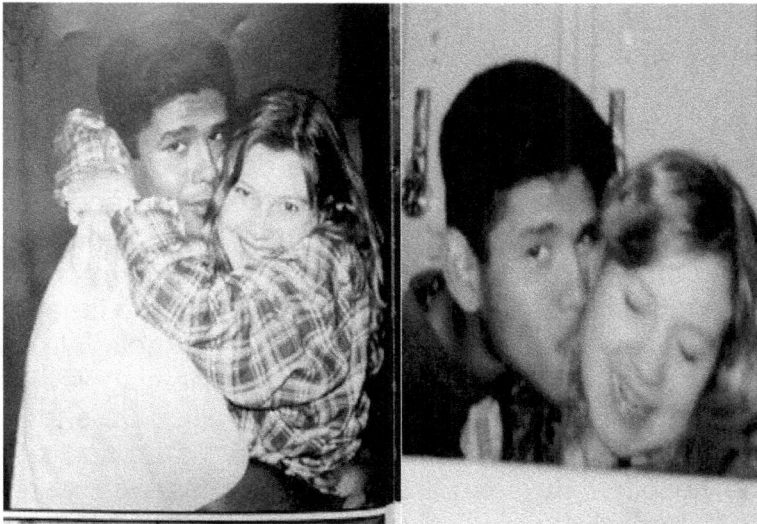

CHAPTER EIGHT

Children and Family during those days....

My children have been through so much. They have written about it. I had to include their own words in this book.

Sydnee~

I was up that night and late and all of a sudden I saw my mom's room light come on and hear her saying I feel like I've been in a car wreck I need to go to Heidi, my neighbor's house, and I saw her walking to the door. So, I helped and my dad took over and followed her to the house and I stayed to make sure Alyssa is still asleep then I see red and blue light out the window, I looked out and I saw my mom being taken out on a gurney to an ambulance I have no idea what's going on but I hope she is okay. I got knots all in my stomach, that feeling you get when something is wrong. Right when I go to check on my sister make sure she is still asleep my dad comes in the door to pick us up and take us to the hospital. He says they think she has overdose or it was maybe something else that they can't find at the moment so they did some tests found that she was bleeding from the back of the head and they call it an " Aneurysm." So, they are going to care flight her to a different hospital because the right Doctor wasn't on duty. When I heard care flight I knew it was bad. It was silent the whole ride to the hospital, we even beat the helicopter to the hospital. We were in the waiting room when my dad told me and my sister this moment will change our lives forever. Basically, the TALK if mom didn't make it. A doctor comes out and says "she's in surgery and she may not make it out this surgery. You need to call any family now" Feeling the tears fall down my cheeks I was thinking the impossible that I could lose my only mom that I have. I just hugged my sister and my dad while we all cried. My life without my mom won't be the same. My mom is my rock my shoulder. All throughout the waiting room you could just hear air conditioning. My dad was reading online about aneurysms and had to call my Nana(Debbie) and Papa (Adrian) and all other close family we have. And Seeing him break down makes me break down even more. I'm just praying and hoping for the best and that she makes the surgery. A Doctor came to talk to dad, my sister and I got so quiet. It was an update on the surgery. The doctor told us "surgery is done and she stable and very swollen.... y'all are able to see her now." He takes us to her room I was the first to go in and I saw my mom in bed just lying there all swollen...I've never seen her like this before. Our lives are forever changed. I'm no longer a regular 15-year-old. I'm a 15-year-old with a life no other teen would ever want. I'm not so sure how I was that strong to handle all that happened. I'm just thankful that she is still in my life no matter if she can't walk straight or if she wobbles. I will love her no matter what. She will be my forever survived super mom!!

Alyssa~

I was sleeping very good when I woke up to my dad coming in the house telling me we need to hurry and get dressed and go to the hospital mom has been taken by care flight and we got to go. "What happened?" "Mom is having an aneurysm very serious." All I could think about was omg my mom was fine today what happened. We left for the hospital.

I think I constantly looked at the sky wondering if what I saw was her or just a plane or helicopter. It was silent in the truck. My sister kept telling me it's going to be ok that mom was strong and can beat this. After what seemed like forever we got to the hospital and come to find out we beat the helicopter there. We heard the helicopter land but they rushed my mom right into surgery so I didn't get to see her. My dad then took my sisters and my hand. We went to the waiting room. My dad told us that from this moment on our lives will change. Mom may not make it through this. Tears just started pouring out my eyes. I can't be without my mom. She is my best friend. My sister and I just looked at each other and became one it felt like. We both looked at dad and nodded, yes dad we understand and we will get through this. We all sat together and prayed. It was silent in that waiting room. Not one word was spoken. Just sniffles. Thoughts of my mom ran through my head. God, I hope she is ok.

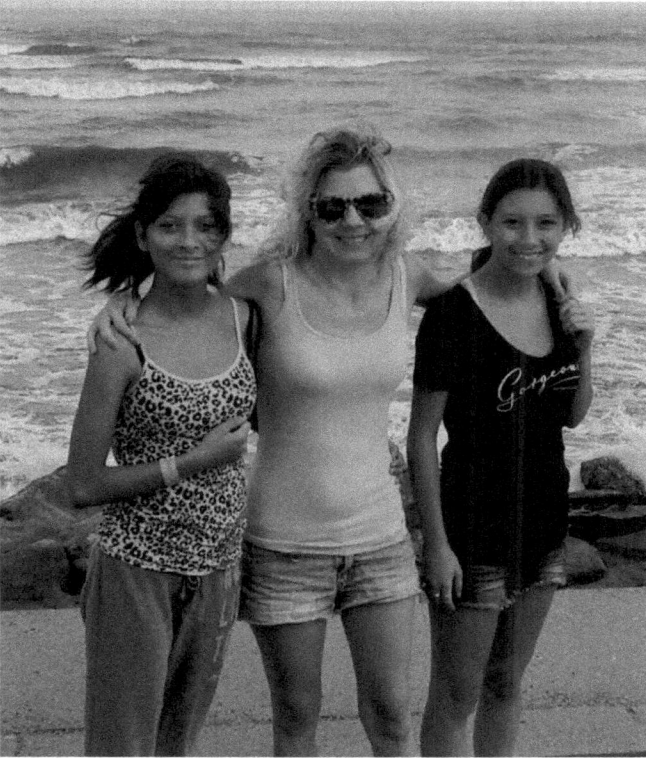

KNOWLEDGE IS POWER
Everything you may not know about AVM's

This is a wonderful quick course provided by the American Heart Association.

What is a brain AVM?

Normally, **arteries** carry blood containing oxygen from the heart to the brain, and **veins** carry blood with less oxygen away from the brain and back to the heart. When an **arteriovenous malformation (AVM)** occurs, a tangle of blood vessels in the brain or on its surface bypasses normal brain tissue and directly diverts blood from the arteries to the veins.

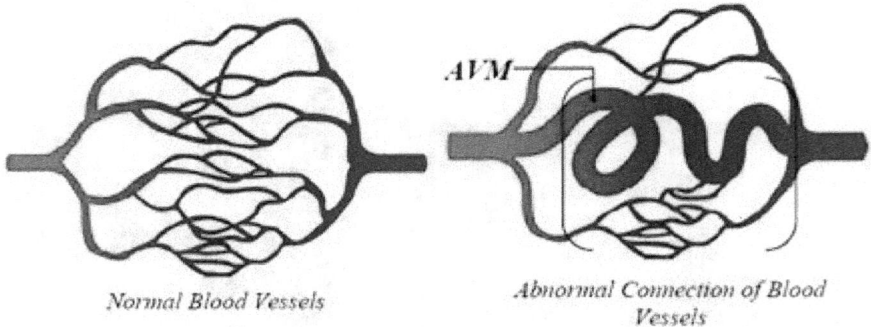

Normal Blood Vessels

Abnormal Connection of Blood Vessels

How common are brain AVMs?

Brain AVMs occur in less than 1 percent of the general population. It's estimated that about one in 200–500 people may have an AVM. AVMs are more common in males than in females.

Why do brain AVMs occur?

We don't know why AVMs occur. Brain AVMs are usually congenital, meaning someone is born with one. But they're usually not hereditary. People probably don't inherit an AVM from their parents, and they probably won't pass one on to their children.

Where do brain AVMs occur?

Brain AVMs can occur anywhere within the brain or on its covering. This includes the four major lobes of the front part of the brain (frontal, parietal, temporal, occipital), the back part of the brain (cerebellum), the brainstem, or the ventricles (deep spaces within the brain that produce and circulate the cerebrospinal fluid).

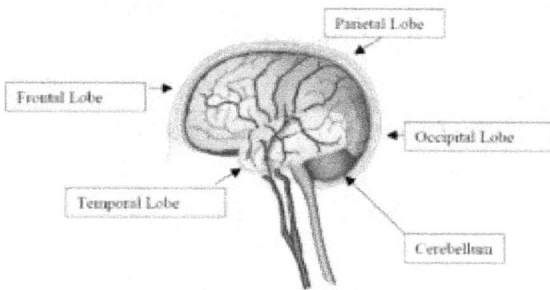

Do brain AVMs change or grow?

Most AVMs don't grow or change much, although the vessels involved may dilate (widen). Some AVMs may shrink due to clots in part of the AVM. Some may enlarge to redirect blood in adjacent vessels toward an AVM.

What are the symptoms of a brain AVM?

Symptoms may vary depending on where the AVM is located:

- More than 50 percent of patients with an AVM have an intracranial hemorrhage.

- Among AVM patients, 20 percent to 25 percent have focal or generalized seizures.
- Patients may have localized pain in the head due to increased blood flow around an AVM.
- Fifteen percent may have difficulty with movement, speech and vision.

What causes brain AVMs to bleed?

A brain AVM contains abnormal and, therefore, "weakened" blood vessels that direct blood away from normal brain tissue. These abnormal and weak blood vessels dilate over time. Eventually they may burst from the high pressure of blood flow from the arteries, causing bleeding into the brain.

What are the chances of a brain AVM bleeding?

The chance of a brain AVM bleeding is 1 percent to 3 percent per year. Over 15 years, the total chance of an AVM bleeding into the brain – causing brain damage and stroke – is 25 percent.

Does one bleed increase the chance of a second bleed?

The risk of recurrent intracranial bleeding is slightly higher for a short time after the first bleed. In two studies, the risk during the first year after initial bleeding was 6 percent and then dropped to the baseline rate. In another study, the risk of recurrence during the first year was 17.9 percent. The risk of recurrent bleeding may be even higher in the first year after the second bleed and has been reported to be 25 percent during that year. People who are between 11 to 35 years old and who have an AVM are at a slightly higher risk of bleeding.

What can happen if a brain AVM causes a bleed?

The risk of death related to each bleed is 10 percent to 15 percent. The chance of permanent brain damage is 20 percent to 30 percent. Each time blood leaks into the brain, normal brain tissue is damaged. This results in loss of normal function, which may be temporary or permanent. Some possible symptoms include arm or leg weakness/paralysis, or difficulty with speech, vision or memory. The amount of brain damage depends on how much blood has leaked from the AVM.

What functions does an AVM affect?

If an AVM bleeds, it can affect one or more normal body functions, depending on the location and extent of the brain injury. Different locations in the brain control different functions:

- Frontal lobe controls personality.
- Parietal lobe controls movement of the arms and legs.
- Temporal lobe controls speech, memory and understanding.
- Occipital lobe controls vision.
- The cerebellum controls walking and coordination.
- Ventricles control the secretion of cerebrospinal fluid.

- The brainstem controls the pathways from all of the above functions to the rest of the body.

Are there different types of brain AVMs?

All blood vessel malformations involving the brain and its surrounding structures are commonly referred to as AVMs. But several types exist:

- **True arteriovenous malformation (AVM).** This is the most common brain vascular malformation. It consists of a tangle of abnormal vessels connecting arteries and veins with no normal intervening brain tissue.
- **Occult or cryptic AVM or cavernous malformations.** This is a vascular malformation in the brain that doesn't actively divert large amounts of blood. It may bleed and often produce seizures.
- **Venous malformation.** This is an abnormality only of the veins. The veins are either enlarged or appear in abnormal locations within the brain.
- **Hemangioma.** These are abnormal blood vessel structures usually found at the surface of the brain and on the skin or facial structures. These represent large and abnormal pockets of blood within normal tissue planes of the body.
- **Dural fistula.** The covering of the brain is called the "dura mater." An abnormal connection between blood vessels that involve only this covering is called a dural fistula. Dural fistulas can occur in any part of the brain

covering. Three kinds of dural fistulas are:
- **Dural carotid cavernous sinus fistula.** These occur behind the eye and usually cause symptoms because they divert too much blood   toward the eye. Patients have eye swelling, decreased vision, redness and congestion of the eye. They often can hear a "swishing" noise.
- **Transverse-Sigmoid sinus dural fistula.** These occur behind the ear. Patients usually complain of hearing a continuous noise (bruit) that occurs with each heartbeat, local pain behind the ear, headaches and neck pain.
- **Sagittal sinus and scalp dural fistula.** These occur toward the top of the head. Patients complain of noise (bruit), headaches, and pain near the top of the head; they may have prominent blood vessels on the scalp and above the ear.

What is the best treatment for a dural fistula?

The best treatment is usually endovascular surgical blocking of the abnormal connections that have caused the fistula. This involves guiding small tubes (catheters) inside the blood vessel with X-ray guidance and blocking off the abnormal connections. Depending on the location and size, many of these can be treated and cured by these less invasive endovascular techniques.

How are AVMs diagnosed?

Most AVMs are detected with either a computed tomography (CT) brain scan or a magnetic resonance imaging (MRI) brain scan. These tests are very good at detecting brain AVMs. They also provide information about the location and size of the AVM and whether it may have bled. A doctor may also perform a cerebral angiogram. This test involves inserting a catheter (small tube) through an artery in the leg (groin). Then it's guided into each of the vessels in the neck going to the brain, and a contrast material (dye) is injected and pictures are taken of all the blood vessels in the brain. For any type of treatment involving an AVM, an angiogram may be needed to better identify the type of AVM.

What factors influence whether an AVM should be treated?

In general, an AVM may be considered for treatment if it has bled, if it's in an area of the brain that can be easily treated and if it's not too large.

What is the best treatment for an AVM?

It depends on what type it is, the symptoms it may be causing and its location and size.

What different types of treatment are available?

- **Medical therapy.** If there are no symptoms or almost none, or if an AVM is in an area of the brain that can't be easily treated, conservative medical management may be indicated. If possible, a person with an AVM should avoid any activities that may excessively elevate blood pressure, such as heavy lifting or straining, and avoid blood thinners like warfarin. A person with an AVM should have regular checkups with a neurologist or neurosurgeon.

- **Surgery.** If an AVM has bled and/or is in an area that can be easily operated upon, then surgical removal may be recommended. The patient is put to sleep with anesthesia, a portion of the skull is removed, and the AVM is surgically removed. When the AVM is completely taken out, the possibility of any further bleeding should be eliminated.
- **Stereotactic radiosurgery.** An AVM that's not too large, but is in an area that's difficult to reach by regular surgery, may be treated with stereotactic radiosurgery. In this procedure, a cerebral angiogram is done to localize the AVM. Focused-beam high energy sources are then concentrated on the brain AVM to produce direct damage to the vessels that will cause a scar and allow the AVM to "clot off."
- **Interventional neuroradiology/endovascular neurosurgery.** It may be possible to treat part or all of the AVM by placing a catheter (small tube) inside the blood vessels that supply the AVM and blocking off the abnormal blood vessels with various materials. These include liquid tissue adhesives (glues), micro coils, particles and other materials used to stop blood flowing to the AVM. The best treatment depends on the symptoms the patient is

having, what type of AVM is present and the AVM's size and location.

What doctors specialize in treating brain AVMs?

- **Vascular neurosurgeons** specialize in surgically removing brain AVMs.
- **Radiation therapists/neurosurgeons** specialize in the stereotactic radiosurgery treatment of brain AVMs.
- **Interventional neuroradiologists/endovascular neurosurgeons** specialize in the endovascular therapy of brain AVMs.
- **Stroke neurologists** specialize in the medical management of brain AVMs.

Neuroradiologists specialize in the diagnosis and imaging of the head, neck, brain and spinal cord. They perform and interpret the CT, MRI, and cerebral angiograms necessary for evaluation, management and treatment. Each of these specialists has had advanced training and is highly skilled at treating complex brain vascular malformations.

The Brain Aneurysm Foundation has also put together some of the most helpful and easy to understand information about Brain Aneurysms.

Brain Aneurysm Basics

Being diagnosed with a brain aneurysm is frightening. Although ruptured aneurysms are relatively uncommon, they represent a very serious illness which is associated with a high rate of mortality and disability. Having survived a ruptured aneurysm is a very difficult experience to have gone through and can be extremely unsettling. Gathering information about your condition can help ease this fear, help begin the healing process, and help bring a sense of comfort and support during a trying time.

What is a brain aneurysm?

A brain aneurysm,

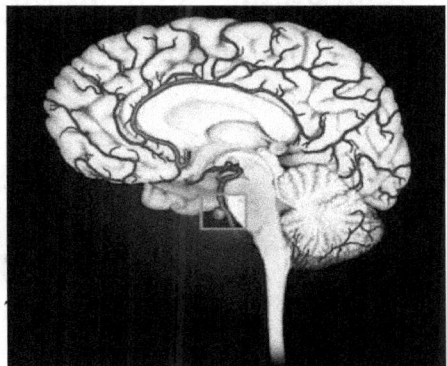

also referred to as a **cerebral aneurysm** or intracranial aneurysm (IA), is a weak bulging spot on the wall of a brain artery very much like a thin balloon or weak spot on an inner tube. Over time, the blood flow within the artery pounds against the thinned portion of the wall and aneurysms form silently from wear and tear on the arteries. As the artery wall becomes gradually thinner from the dilation, the blood flow causes the weakened wall to swell outward. This pressure may cause the aneurysm to rupture and allow blood to escape into the space around the brain. A ruptured brain aneurysm commonly requires advanced surgical treatment.

What are the two types of aneurysms?

Saccular

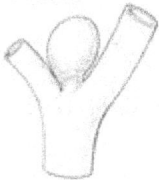

A saccular aneurysm is the most common type of aneurysm and account for 80% to 90% of all intracranial aneurysms and are the most common cause of nontraumatic **subarachnoid hemorrhage (SAH)**. It is also known as a "berry" aneurysm because of its shape. The berry aneurysm looks like a sac or berry forming at the bifuraction or the "Y" segment of arteries. It has a neck and stem. These small, berry-like projections occur at arterial bifurcations and branches of the large arteries at the base of the brain, known as the **Circle of Willis**.

The **fusiform aneurysm** is a less common type of aneurysm. It looks like an outpouching of an arterial wall on both sides of the artery or like a blood vessel that is expanded in all directions. The fusiform aneurysm does not have a stem and it seldom ruptures.

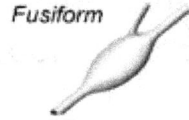

Fusiform

Understanding the Brain

To understand aneurysms, it is helpful to understand the circulatory system of the brain. The heart pumps oxygen- and nutrient-laden blood to the brain, face, and scalp via two major sets of vessels: the internal carotid arteries and the vertebral arteries. The jugular and other veins bring blood out of the brain.

The carotid arteries run along the front of the neck - one on the left and one on the right. They are what you feel when you take your pulse just under your jaw. The carotid arteries split into external and internal arteries near the top of the neck.

The external carotid arteries supply blood to the

face and scalp. The internal carotid arteries supply blood to the front (anterior) three-fifths of cerebrum, except for parts of the temporal and occipital lobes.

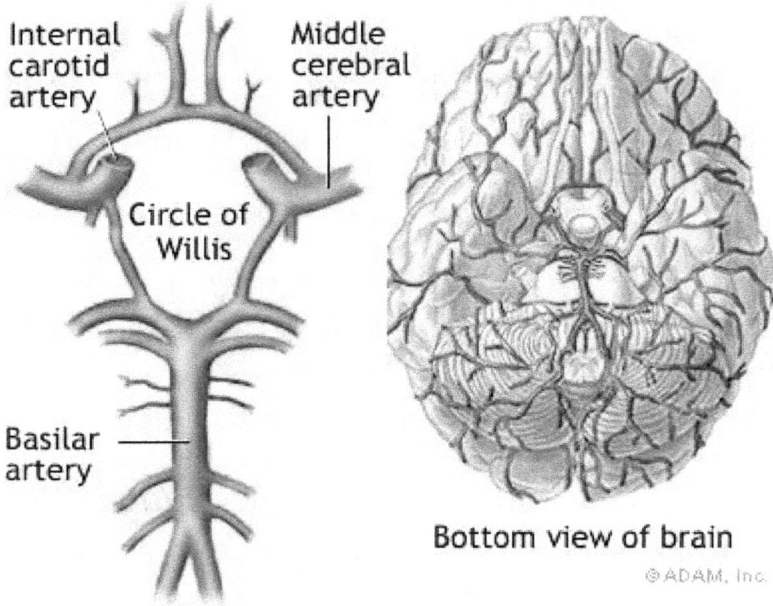

Bottom view of brain

©ADAM, Inc.

The vertebral arteries travel along the spinal column and cannot be felt from the outside. They join to form a single basilar artery (hence the name vertebrobasilar arteries) near the brain stem at the base of the skull. The arteries supply blood to the posterior two-fifths of the cerebrum, part of the cerebellum, and the brain stem.

Because the brain relies on only two sets of major arteries for its blood supply, it is very important that these arteries are healthy. These arteries that conduct blood to the brain — the internal-carotid and vertebral arteries — connect through the Circle of Willis, which loops around the brainstem at the base of the brain. From this circle, other arteries — the anterior cerebral artery (ACA), the middle cerebral artery (MCA), and the posterior cerebral artery (PCA) — arise and travel to all parts of the brain. Brain aneurysms tend to occur at the junctions between the arteries that make up the Circle of Willis.

CIRCLE OF WILLIS

Internal Carotid Artery

Anterior Cerebral Artery

Middle Cerebral Artery

Circle of Willis

Anterior Communicating Artery

Posterior Communicating Artery

Posterior Cerebral Artery

Basilar Artery

Vertebral Artery

Posterior Inferior Cerebellar Artery

WALTER CRANE

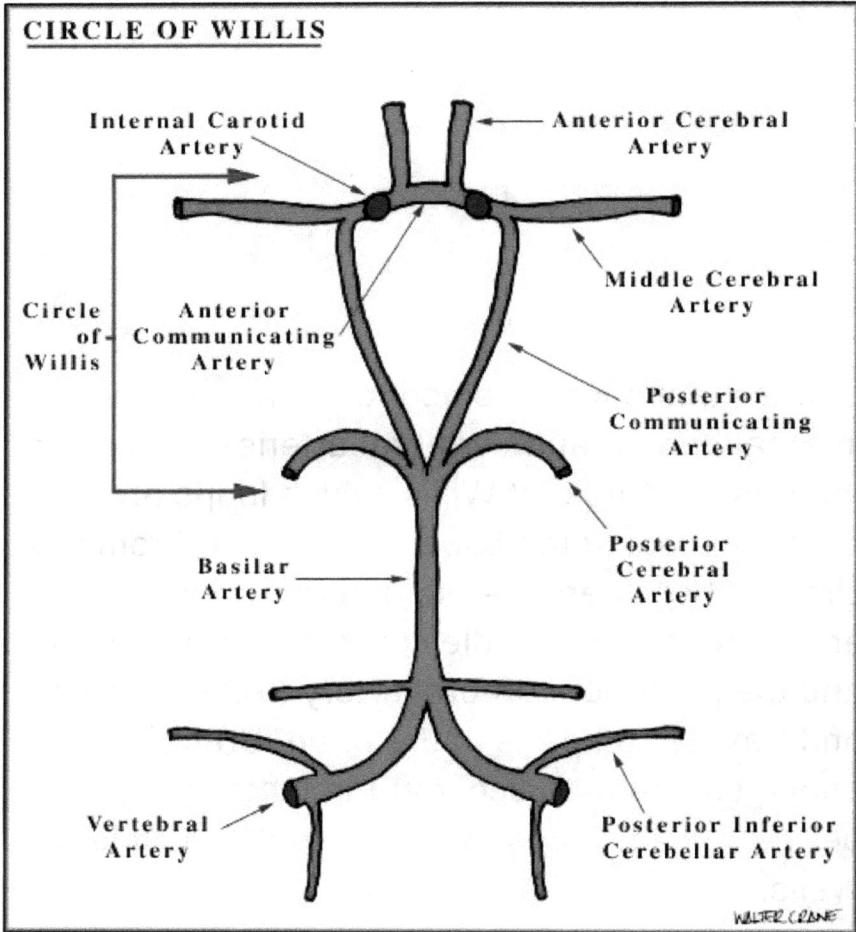

Warning Signs/ Symptoms

Unruptured brain aneurysms are typically completely asymptomatic. These aneurysms are typically small in size, usually less than one half inch in diameter. However, large unruptured aneurysms can occasionally press on the brain or the nerves stemming out of the brain and may result in various neurological symptoms. Any individual experiencing some or all of the following symptoms, regardless of age, should undergo immediate and careful evaluation by a physician.

- Localized Headache
- Dilated pupils
- Blurred or double vision
- Pain above and behind eye
- Weakness and numbness
- Difficulty speaking

Ruptured brain aneurysms usually result in a subarachnoid hemorrhage (SAH), which is defined as bleeding into the subarachnoid space. When blood escapes into the space around the brain, it can cause sudden symptoms.

Seek Medical Attention Immediately If You Are Experiencing Some Or All Of These Symptoms:

- Sudden severe headache, the worst headache of your life
- Loss of consciousness
- Nausea/Vomiting
- Stiff Neck
- Sudden blurred or double vision
- Sudden pain above/behind the eye or difficulty seeing
- Sudden change in mental status/awareness
- Sudden trouble walking or dizziness
- Sudden weakness and numbness
- Sensitivity to light (photophobia)
- Seizure

• Drooping eyelids

Brain Aneurysm Statistics and Facts

✓ An estimated 6 million people in the United States have an unruptured brain aneurysm, or 1 in 50 people.

✓ The annual rate of rupture is approximately 8 - 10 per 100,000 people or about 30,000 people in the United States suffer a brain aneurysm rupture. There is a brain aneurysm rupturing every 18 minutes. Ruptured brain aneurysms are fatal in about 40% of cases. Of those who survive, about 66% suffer some permanent neurological deficit.

✓ Approximately 15% of patients with aneurysmal subarachnoid hemorrhage (SAH) die before reaching the hospital. Most of the deaths from subarachnoid hemorrhage are due to rapid and massive brain injury from the initial bleeding which is not correctable by medical and surgical interventions.

✓ 4 out of 7 people who recover from a ruptured brain aneurysm will have disabilities.

✓ Brain aneurysms are most prevalent in people ages 35 - 60, but can occur in children as well. The median age when aneurysmal **hemorrhagic stroke** occurs is 50 years old and there are typically no warning signs. Most aneurysms develop after the age of 40.

✓ Most aneurysms are small, about 1/8 inch to nearly one inch, and an estimated 50 to 80 percent of all aneurysms do not rupture during the course of a person's lifetime. Aneurysms larger than one inch are referred to as "giant" aneurysms and can pose a particularly high risk and can be difficult to treat.

✓ Women, more than men, suffer from brain aneurysms at a ratio of 3:2.

✓ Ruptured brain aneurysms account for 3 - 5% of all new strokes.

✓ Subarachnoid hemorrhage (SAH) is one of the most feared causes of acute headache upon presentation to the emergency department. Headache accounts for 1 - 2% of the emergency room visits and up to 4% of visits to the primary care offices. Among all the patients who present to the emergency room with headaches, approximately 1% has subarachnoid hemorrhage. One study put the figure at 4%.

✓ Accurate early diagnosis is critical, as the initial hemorrhage may be fatal, may result in devastating neurologic outcomes, or may produce minor symptoms. Despite widespread neuroimaging availability, misdiagnosis or delays in diagnosis occurs in up to 25% of patients with subarachnoid hemorrhage (SAH) when initially presenting for medical treatment. Failure to do a scan results in 73% of these misdiagnoses. This makes SAH a low-frequency, high-risk disease.

✓ There are almost 500,000 deaths worldwide each year caused by brain aneurysms and half the victims are younger than 50.

✓ Based on a 2004 study, the combined lost wages of survivors of brain aneurysm rupture and their caretaker for a year were $138,000,000

✓ The cost of a brain aneurysm treated by clipping via open brain surgery more than doubles in cost after the aneurysm has ruptured. The cost of a brain aneurysm treated by coiling, which is less invasive and is done through a **catheter**, increases by about 70% after the aneurysm has ruptured.

✓ 10 - 15% of patients diagnosed with a brain aneurysm will harbor more than one aneurysm

Risk Factors

Risk factors that doctors and researchers believe contribute to the formation of brain aneurysms:

✓ Smoking
✓ High blood pressure or hypertension
✓ Congenital resulting from inborn abnormality in artery wall
✓ Family history of brain aneurysms
✓ Age over 40
✓ Gender, women compared with men have an increased incidence of aneurysms at a ratio of 3:2

✓ Other disorders: Ehlers-Danlos Syndrome, Polycystic Kidney Disease, Marfan Syndrome, and Fibromuscular Dysplasia(FMD)
   ✓ Presence arteriovenous malformation
   ✓ Drug use, particularly cocaine
   ✓ Infection
   ✓ Tumors
   ✓ Traumatic head injury
   ✓ Risk factors that doctors and researchers believe contribute to the rupture of brain aneurysms:
   ✓ Smoking
   ✓ High blood pressure or hypertension

BRAIN INJURY~ THE STAGES OF RECOVERY

What happens to the brain during injury and the early stages of recovery from TBI?

What is a brain injury?

Traumatic brain injury (TBI) refers to damage to the brain caused by an external physical force such as a car accident, a gunshot wound to the head, or a fall. A TBI is not caused by something internal such as a stroke or tumor, and does not include damage to the brain due to prolonged lack of oxygen (anoxic brain injuries). It is possible to have a TBI and never lose consciousness. For example, someone with a penetrating gunshot wound to the head may not lose consciousness.

Commonly accepted criteria established by the **TBI Model Systems (TBIMS)** to identify the presence and severity of TBI include:

Damage to brain tissue caused by an external force and at least one of the following:

- A documented loss of consciousness
- The person cannot recall the actual traumatic event (amnesia)
- The person has a skull fracture, post-traumatic seizure, or an abnormal brain scan due to the trauma

Causes of TBI

Statistics from Centers for Disease Control for 2002-2006 indicate that the leading cause of brain injury is falls (35%) followed by car crashes (17%) and being struck by an object (16%). Emergency room visits due to TBI caused by falls are increasing for both younger and older people. However, if you focus only on moderate to severe TBI (those injuries that require admission to a neurointensive care unit), car crashes are the most frequent cause of TBI, followed by gunshot wound, falls, and assault.

Types of injuries

The brain is about 3.4 pounds of extremely delicate soft tissue floating in fluid within the skull. Under the skull there are three layers of membrane that cover and protect the brain. The brain tissue is soft and therefore can be compressed (squeezed), pulled, and stretched. When there is sudden speeding up and slowing down, such as in a car crash or fall, the brain can move around violently inside the skull, resulting in injury.

Closed versus open head injury

Closed means the skull and brain contents have not been penetrated (broken into or through), whereas *open* means the skull and other protective layers are penetrated and exposed to air. A classic example of an open head injury is a gunshot wound to the head. A classic closed head injury is one that occurs as the result of a motor vehicle crash.

In a ***closed head injury***, damage occurs because of a blow to the person's head or having the head stop suddenly after moving at high speed. This causes the brain to move forward and back or from side to side, such that it collides with the bony skull around it. This jarring movement bruises brain tissue, damages axons (part of the nerve cell), and tears blood vessels. After a closed head injury, damage can occur in specific brain areas (localized injury) or throughout the brain (diffuse axonal injury).

Damage following ***open head injury*** tends to be localized and therefore damage tends to be limited to a specific area of the brain. However, such injuries can be as severe as closed head injuries, depending on the destructive path of the bullet or other invasive object within the brain.

Primary versus secondary injuries

Primary injuries occur at the time of injury and there is nothing that physicians can do to reverse those injuries. Instead, the goal of the treatment team in the hospital is to prevent any further, or secondary, injury to the brain. Below are some primary injuries.

✓ ***Skull fracture*** occurs when there is a breaking or denting of the skull. Pieces of bone pressing on the brain can cause injury, often referred to as a depressed skull fracture.

✓ *Localized injury* means that a particular area of the brain is injured. Injuries can involve bruising (contusions) or bleeding (hemorrhages) on the surface of or within any layer of the brain.

✓ *Diffuse axonal Injury* (DAI) involves damage throughout the brain and loss of consciousness. DAI is a stretching injury to the neurons (the cell bodies of the brain) and axons (fibers that allow for communication from one neuron to another neuron). Everything our brains do for us depends on neurons communicating. When the brain is injured, axons can be pulled, stretched, and torn. If there is too much injury to the axon, the neuron will not survive. In a DAI, this happens to neurons all over the brain. This type of damage is often difficult to detect with brain scans.

Secondary injuries occur after the initial injury, usually within a few days. Secondary injury may be caused by oxygen not reaching the brain, which can be the result of continued low blood pressure or increased intracranial pressure (pressure inside the skull) from brain tissue swelling.

Measuring the severity of TBI

Severity of injury refers to the degree or extent of brain tissue damage. The degree of damage is estimated by measuring the duration of loss of consciousness, the depth of coma and level of amnesia (memory loss), and through brain scans.

The *Glasgow Coma Scale* (GCS) is used to

measure the depth of coma. The GCS rates three aspects of functioning: eye opening, movement and verbal response. Individuals in deep coma score very low on all these aspects of functioning, while those less severely injured or recovering from coma score higher. A GCS score of 3 indicates the deepest level of coma, describing a person who is totally unresponsive. A score of 9 or more indicates that the person is no longer in coma, but is not fully alert. The highest score (15) refers to a person who is fully conscious.

A person's first GCS score is often done at the roadside by the emergency response personnel. In many instances, moderately to severely injured people are intubated (a tube is placed down the throat and into the air passage into the lungs) at the scene of the injury to ensure the person gets enough oxygen. To do the intubation the person must be sedated (given medication that makes the person go to sleep). So, by the time the person arrives at the hospital he/she has already received sedating medications and has a breathing tube in place. Under these conditions it is impossible for a person to talk, so the doctors cannot assess the verbal part of the GCS. People in this situation often receive a T after the GCS score, indicating that they were intubated when the examination took place, so you might see a score of 5T, for instance. The GCS is done at intervals in the neurointensive care unit to document a person's recovery.

Post-traumatic amnesia (PTA) is another good estimate for severity of a brain injury. Anytime a person has a major blow to the head he or she will not remember the injury and related events for some time afterward. People with these injuries might not recall having spoken to someone just a couple of hours ago and may repeat things they have already said. This is the period of posttraumatic amnesia. The longer the duration of amnesia, the more severe the brain damage.

CT or MRI Scan Results

The cranial tomography (CT) scan is a type of X-ray that shows problems in the brain such as bruises, blood clots, and swelling. CT scans are not painful. People with moderate to severe TBI will have several CT scans while in the hospital to keep track of lesions (damaged areas in the brain). In some cases, a magnetic resonance imaging (MRI) scan may also be performed. This also creates a picture of the brain based on magnetic properties of molecules in tissue. Most people with severe TBI will have an abnormality on a CT scan or MRI scan. These scans cannot detect all types of brain injuries, so it is possible to have a severe TBI and be in coma even though the scan results are normal.

Brain tissue response to injury

Common Problems:

Increased intracranial pressure

The brain is like any other body tissue when it gets injured: it fills with fluid and swells. Because of the hard skull around it, however, the brain has nowhere to expand as it swells. This swelling increases pressure inside the head (intracranial pressure), which can cause further injury to the brain. Decreasing and controlling intracranial pressure is a major focus of medical treatment early after a TBI. If intracranial pressure remains high, it can prevent blood passage to tissue, which results in further brain injury.

Neurochemical problems that disrupt functioning

Our brains operate based on a delicate chemistry. Chemical substances in the brain called neurotransmitters are necessary for communication between neurons, the specialized cells within our central nervous system. When the brain is functioning normally, chemical signals are sent from neuron to neuron, and groups of neurons work together to perform functions.

TBI disturbs the delicate chemistry of the brain so that the neurons cannot function normally. This results in changes in thinking and behavior. It can take weeks and sometimes months for the brain to resolve the chemical imbalance that occurs with TBI. As the chemistry of the brain improves, so can the person's ability to function. This is one reason that someone may make rapid progress in the first few weeks after an injury.

Natural plasticity (ability of change) of the brain

The brain is a dynamic organ that has a natural ability to adapt and change with time. Even after it has been injured, the brain changes by setting up new connections between neurons that carry the messages within our brains. We now know the brain can create new neurons in some parts of the brain, although the extent and purpose of this is still uncertain.

Plasticity of the brain occurs at every stage of development throughout the life cycle. Plasticity is more likely to occur when there is stimulation of the neural system, meaning that the brain must be active to adapt. Changes do not occur without exposure to a stimulating environment that prompts the brain to work. These changes do not occur quickly. That is one of the reasons that recovery goes on for months and sometimes years following TBI.

Rehabilitation sets in motion the process of adaptation and change. Keep in mind that formal rehabilitation, such as received in a hospital from professional therapists, is a good initial step, but in most cases this must be followed by outpatient therapies and stimulating activities in the injured person's home.

What is the TBIMS?

The TBIMS is a group of 16 medical centers funded by the National Institute on Disability and Rehabilitation Research (NIDRR). The TBIMS works to maintain and improve a cost-effective, comprehensive service delivery system for people who experience a TBI, from the moment of their injury and throughout their life span.

Common stages

In the first few weeks after a brain injury, swelling, bleeding or changes in brain chemistry often affect the function of healthy brain tissue. The injured person's eyes may remain closed, and the person may not show signs of awareness. As swelling decreases and blood flow and brain chemistry improve, brain function usually improves. With time, the person's eyes may open, sleep-wake cycles may begin, and the injured person may follow commands, respond to family members, and speak. Some terms that might be used in these early stages of recovery are:

  ✓ Coma: The person is unconscious, does not respond to visual stimulation or sounds, and is unable to communicate or show emotional responses.
  ✓ Vegetative State: The person has sleep-wake cycles, and startles or briefly orients to visual stimulation and sounds.
  ✓ Minimally Conscious State: The person is partially conscious, knows where sounds and visual stimulation are coming from, reaches for objects, responds to commands now and then, can vocalize at times, and shows emotion.

A period of confusion and disorientation often follows a TBI. A person's ability to pay attention and learn stops, and agitation, nervousness, restlessness or frustration may appear. Sleeping patterns may be disrupted. The person may overreact to stimulation and become physically aggressive. This stage can be disturbing for family because the person behaves so uncharacteristically.

Inconsistent behavior is also common. Some days are better than others. For example, a person may begin to follow a command (lift your leg, squeeze my finger) and then not do so again for a time. This stage of recovery may last days or even weeks for some. In this stage of recovery, try not to become anxious about inconsistent signs of progress. Ups and downs are normal.

Later stages of recovery can bring increased

brain and physical function. The person's ability to respond may improve gradually.

Length of recovery

The fastest improvement happens in about the first six months after injury. During this time, the injured person will likely show many improvements and may seem to be steadily getting better. The person continues to improve between six months and two years after injury, but this varies for different people and may not happen as fast as the first six months. Improvements slow down substantially after two years but may still occur many years after injury. Most people continue to have some problems, although they may not be as bad as they were early after injury. Rate of improvement varies from person to person.

Long-term impacts

It is common and understandable for family members to have many questions about the long-term effects of the brain injury on the injured person's ability to function in the future. Unfortunately, it is difficult to determine the long-term effects for many reasons.

   ✓ First, brain injury is a relatively new area of treatment and research. We have only begun to understand the long-term effects in patients one, five, and ten years after injury.
   ✓ Brain scans and other tests are not always able to show the extent of the injury, so it is sometimes difficult early on to fully understand how serious the injury is.

✓ The type of brain injury and extent of secondary problems such as brain swelling varies a great deal from person to person.

✓ Age and pre-injury abilities also affect how well a person will recover.

We do know that the more severe the injury the less likely the person will fully recover. The length of time a person remains in a coma and duration of loss of memory (amnesia) following the coma are useful in predicting how well a person will recover.

The Rancho Los Amigos Levels of Cognitive Functioning (RLCF) is one of the best and most widely used ways of describing recovery from brain injury. The RLCF describes ten levels of cognitive (thinking) recovery. Research has shown that the speed at which a person progresses through the levels of the RLCF can predict how fully a person will recover.

The Rancho Los Amigos Levels of Cognitive Functioning

Level 1-- No Response: Person appears to be in a deep sleep.

Level 2-- Generalized Response: Person reacts inconsistently and not directly in response to stimuli.

Level 3-- Localized Response: Person reacts inconsistently and directly to stimuli.

Level 4-- Confused/Agitated: Person is extremely agitated and confused.

Level 5-- Confused-Inappropriate/Non-agitated: Person is confused and responses to commands are inaccurate.

Level 6-- Confused-Appropriate: Person is confused and responds accurately to commands.

Level 7-- Automatic-Appropriate: Person can go through daily routine with minimal to no confusion.

Level 8-- Purposeful-Appropriate: Person has functioning memory, and is aware of and responsive to their environment.

Level 9-- Purposeful-Appropriate: Person can go through daily routine while aware of need for stand by assistance.

Level 10-- Purposeful-Appropriate/Modified Independent: Person can go through daily routine but may require more time or compensatory strategies.

Recovery two years after brain injury

Based on information of people with moderate to severe TBI who received acute medical care and inpatient rehabilitation services at a TBI Model System, two years post-injury:

- Most people continue to show decreases in disability.
- 34% of people required some level of supervision during the day and/or night.
- 93% of people are living in a private residence.
- 34% are living with their spouse or significant other; 29% are living with their parents.

- 33% are employed; 29% are unemployed; 26% are retired due to any reason; and 3% are students.

Disclaimer

This information is not meant to replace the advice from a medical professional. You should consult your health care provider regarding specific medical concerns or treatment.

Source

This health information content is based on research evidence whenever available and represents the consensus of expert opinion of the TBI Model Systems directors.

Our health information content is based on research evidence and/or professional consensus and has been reviewed and approved by an editorial team of experts from the TBI Model Systems.

Authorship

Understanding TBI was developed by Thomas Novack, PhD and Tamara Bushnik, PhD in collaboration with the Model System Knowledge Translation Center. Portions of this document were adapted from materials developed by the Mayo Clinic TBIMS, Baylor Institute for Rehabilitation, and from Picking up the pieces after TBI: A guide for Family Members, by Angelle M. Sander, PhD, Baylor College of Medicine (2002).

POSITIVE

I wake up on a positive side as much as possible these days. I wasn't always like this, but after my AVM I believe one small positive thing in the morning can make your day a great one. Before my AVM I wasn't such a positive thinker, but after the incident I started focusing on the things that could go right instead of wrong. I still stress even more easily now so this is important that I start my day as positive as possible so hopefully the whole day is as wonderful as a field of sunflowers.

Thinking about that I realize I took many things for granted before that now I don't. Waking up breathing every day! You never know when this will end. No natural disaster happened today. Making a peanut butter and jelly sandwich is harder than what you think, I never thought that until I tried making one and now it takes me a good 15 minutes to make one so I tend to enjoy it. My family is alive and healthy, I'm blessed to witness another day by their side. Watching the clouds form and feeling the wind on my face. The other day my daughters and I went to the garden center to get flowers for my garden, it was extremely hot. Out of the blue it started raining. We continued to look and pick out flowers in the rain. The sprinkles touched our face and cooled us off, this was a memorable moment for me. Before my AVM we would have probably darted for cover. Instead we felt Mother Nature and enjoyed. I don't just keep walking by dandelions now I don't see weeds, I see wishes. Enjoying the wonderful taste and flavor of different entries or drinks, in my case, coffee! Feeling the ocean sand between my toes and under my feet while the waves hit against my ankles, getting that sinking sensation. I never really enjoyed my family until after my AVM, don't get me wrong I enjoyed them just not really have those moments. Now I notice those moments and I savor them. I write about them, so hopefully one day they will read my treasured moments with them. For example, feeding the seagulls every Sunday! I used to not care for those rats with wings as a few call them, now I love hearing and watching them enjoy the bread we toss their way. There's so much that goes on in everyone's life, I choose to start my day embracing what I can cause tomorrow is not promised. My family always says," I love you" because they know how easily how things can change in an instant. The fact that no one knows if they may have an aneurysm or an AVM puts everyone at risk, so no one knows when danger may strike. Therefore, we want the other one to know we love them and enjoy our time together.

So many young people in the world experience an aneurysm and don't survive. I'm one of few that has survived. Many call me a blessing and a miracle. I can say I'm blessed to be here today and I see the things that I once took for granted very differently now. Example, a dandelion a weed that so many think is an eye sore. Yet, I see it as a beautiful and so delicate lucky charm just like me.

Today, I am here, I try my hardest to make my light shine on so many others. I can't say why I survived but I can say miracles do happen and I am proof. Many people who have Aneurysms become our angels and watch after us. I got that second chance at life and that fork in my dirt road caused me to go another direction. This dirt road has its ups and downs of course, but no matter where it takes me I will still shine.